The Anomaly

Living Off Donated Organs and Dark Humor

Inka Nisinbnaum

Contents

To Steffi, who always talked about the USA, how Americans call salami "pepperoni" and how much she enjoyed having been there. I never got the chance to tell her about my *America; she died of chronic rejection before I arrived in the States, but every time I order pepperoni pizza for my kid, I think of her.*

And to my donor without whom this book would be filled with nothing but empty pages.

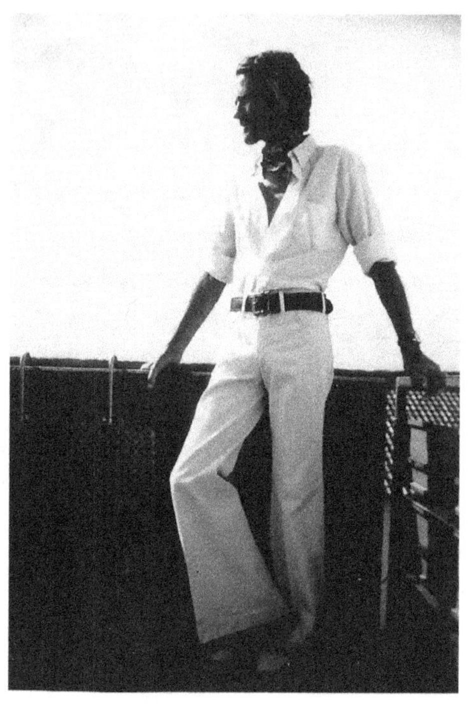

Ingo, summer 1978

1

This Is Bullshit

Death turned on the light at the end of the tunnel, just for me, one day in class. His invitation was imminent—I knew it was. But did he know I was a stubborn one? I could just turn around, flip him the bird, and choose darkness instead. Couldn't I?

I had taken the bus to university, sitting near one of the opened windows, feeling the airstream coming in. Riding my bicycle wasn't an option anymore—too much coughing, too exhausting, and with the bus, I was always on time.

Once I arrived at the lecture hall, lit by humming fluorescent lights and filled with stale air from the '70s, I shuffled over vomit-green linoleum floor and chose a seat in one of the upper rows. It was best for me to sit up, in one of the less crowded rows. If I'd get another coughing fit, I could slip out into the hallway without interrupting the lecture, which was less embarrassing than coughing my lungs out while everyone watched. My classmates' eyes were always like saucers when I coughed.

I started to unpack my things—placing my notepad, pen, and thermos filled with tea onto the tiny desk in front of me where someone had scratched I love psychology into the wood, followed by You need therapy—and watched my fellow students arrive. I suddenly wished I hadn't skipped breakfast, or at least packed a snack. Lately, I just couldn't eat in the morning. No cereal, no toast, not even coffee. I felt hungry and stuffed all the time. But hunger was winning on that day in July.

For a moment, I considered calling out to one of my fellow students three rows below and asking if she had anything to eat in her backpack, but my attempt was cut short as I heard the door close with a deliberate thump. Our professor had arrived.

Everyone sat down in their seats, pens ready, eyes up front. Our professor was not one who accepted anything else but utter silence, and that's when it hit me: *this* was bullshit. Listening to a lecture about educational psychology was bullshit. My skipping breakfast in the morning was bullshit. Everything was bullshit because none of it mattered.

I was dying. Actually dying.

I had known it for a while: acute liver failure. I wasn't surprised by it, not really, but up until this moment, I had always been able to downplay it. I had told myself a million times: *Tomorrow will be better. Tomorrow you will eat more. Maybe even a small cereal in the morning. Liver is a resilient organ; it won't just die on you.* But it was, I just knew it. This was real, and I couldn't sit here and ignore it any longer. I had to do something. I had to forget about educational psychology and save my life instead.

While my professor settled in, I gathered up my things and left, the door closing behind me with an even more deliberate thump.

Outside in the empty hall, I just stood for a moment. Deserted linoleum floor to my right and left, the only sound the muffled words of my professor and the buzzing of the never-ending fluorescent light above me.

I wanted to go home. I wanted to take the bus back to my apartment, close every door there was behind me, and just cry. Full-grown liver cirrhosis was bad. Real bad. And I didn't even earn it by drinking gallons of alcohol partying my life away—no, I had inherited it at birth: the genetic disease called cystic fibrosis, or CF for short. CF is mostly known as a lung disease, and no, my lungs weren't in great shape, either, but as always, I had gotten the shit end of the stick and a failing liver to boot.

Desperately, I wrapped my arms around my body, trying to hold it together. I knew my bus wouldn't arrive for another twenty-five minutes. Twenty-five minutes, plus the ten-minute drive home before I could allow myself to fall apart.

I forced myself to swallow the sour taste in my mouth. I rubbed my eyes to keep any tears hidden, then shook my head.

Don't think about it, I told myself. *Don't think about your dying liver, at least not now. Only once you are home and alone. Not yet, not y—*

A squeaking sound interrupted my thoughts. Shoes on linoleum, no doubt. I looked up to see a business student coming toward me: suit pants (neatly ironed), buttoned shirt, and instead of a backpack, a briefcase—exactly how my business-studying roommate Aria was dressed and exactly the opposite of my worn-down Converse, faded jeans, wrinkly T-shirt, and, of course, a backpack. We exchanged a quick nod when she passed me. I crossed my fingers, hoping she wouldn't stop and ask if I was okay. She didn't. She kept walking until she vanished around the next corner.

Thank God I didn't know her. Any of my fellow students would have stopped and asked if I was okay, would have tried to use some of our newly learned psychology interventions on me, but I had no desire to talk to anyone. First, I myself had to understand what was happening. Was I truly on the brink of dying? Was that even possible when you're only twenty-two years old? Maybe my blood sugar was too low, and that's why I felt weird and not in control. Whatever it was, I didn't want to stand there and embarrass myself any longer. I had to leave and figure this out for myself.

I left the hallway and walked outside, then circled the rectangular red brick building of Clinical Psychology, shaded by tree branches that covered the path. I looked for a place to sit and wait for my bus when I spotted the abandoned basketball court right beside the psychology faculty. I knew immediately no one would find me there because nobody ever used the court. Its hoops were bent, shaped more like ovals, and definitely not wide enough for anyone to score. The court's surface was ripped, like green carpet peeling off the floor, and trash piled up in the corners of the surrounding wire fence. *It looks dead,* I thought as I sat down on a bench.

Just the way I felt.

First thing I did was check my blood sugar. Since age eighteen, I'd had diabetes, another side effect of having CF. Yes, I truly got the golden ticket. If it was too low, it could most definitely be the reason for my doomsday feelings. All kinds of weird thoughts could run through one's mind when blood sugar was dangerously low, but it wasn't. It was perfect: 113.

"*Scheiße.*" Shit.

I shoved everything back in my backpack, closed the zipper, and ground my teeth for a moment, but I couldn't stop my chin from shivering—the tears just started to flow. A Snickers wouldn't be able to save me, after all; it would take more than that, and there was only one cure for a failing liver at the age of twenty-two—a liver transplant—but who had time for a liver transplant these days? I didn't, but of course, life didn't care.

The more I thought about it, the angrier I got. Angry at life, angry that I had to deal with something as big as a solid organ transplant;

angry that I couldn't even go to university without being bothered by my disease, and angry at everyone around me who didn't need an organ transplant. Everyone else who could simply finish their degree, get a job, and live life like it was no big deal.

Except me.

I pulled up my nose, tried to wipe the tears off my face with the short sleeve of my T-shirt, and searched through my backpack and pockets for a tissue or an unused napkin. No such luck.

Life was just brilliant.

The only good thing was that it didn't come as a surprise. I had known for some time that my liver wasn't doing too well. I didn't feel pain, my skin wasn't yellow, but I had a condition called ascites, an unmistakable sign of liver failure. Ascites is nothing more than accumulated liquid in the abdomen, but mine was bad. So bad, my pants were always unbuttoned because my belly didn't fit anymore. The ascites was also the reason for my skipped breakfast in the morning; and of course, the reason I was out of breath most of the time was due to my swollen belly squeezing my lungs. The last time I had been out with a friend dancing at a club, a guy had congratulated me for going out and enjoying my life, despite being pregnant.

I smiled, remembering the stupid expression on his face when I told him I wasn't pregnant but terminally ill. Priceless.

I shook off the memory and pulled up my nose one more time. I tried to rub away the bags I surely had under my eyes from crying and got up to go to my bus stop. Even though I wanted to keep sitting at the abandoned basketball court and pity myself for carrying the load of the world, for being the poorest smug in the universe, I was also stubborn, and especially stubborn when it came to my health. Whenever a doctor told me, "Inka, you will never get that lung function back," or "You will never recover from this," it always sounded to me like a dare

I couldn't turn down. You tell me never, and I'll show you. Same as now. If life wanted to throw sticks between my legs, see me fall, make this personal, I was ready. Bring it on, life. All I needed was a new plan, a new direction to turn to . . . and enough anger to pull me through.

When I arrived home, I opened the door to our sunlit, over one-hundred-years-old apartment and heard the wooden floorboards creak under the paws of my skinny sighthound Fenja. Then everything fell off me: my backpack, my keys, my desperation, my self-pity.

I suddenly knew what I had to do. I had a plan.

When I was ten years old, I had decided to earn an entry in the *Guinness Book of World Records* for being the oldest CF patient who ever lived. *Now*, since I knew I needed a new liver, since I knew there was no way around an organ transplant, I would become the oldest living liver transplant recipient instead.

"I'll show you!" I yelled at the empty apartment, because anger was easier to deal with than despair.

But even though it felt great hiding my actual emotions under a layer of anger and behind a ridiculous new plan, I wasn't going to decide anything without talking to the people who had fought for my life from day one: my parents. I quickly (and finally) ate breakfast, packed a few things, grabbed my dog Fenja, and jumped into my car.

I was on my way to see my parents.

Back then in 2001, I still lived in Northern Germany, where the land was flat, the people straightforward, and the food a mixture of Pinkel (sausage with groats) served with kale and small shrimp bread rolls. My university was in Oldenburg, the capital of Pinkel sausages, which lies a hundred miles west of Hamburg, and two hundred miles north of Düsseldorf, where my parents lived. Düsseldorf is a rather big town in the Lower Rhine region, known for its international business and financial center, fashion, modern architecture, and its rivalry with Cologne, only thirty miles south of it.

Outside of locals, no one would know about the rivalry unless they ordered the wrong beer in the wrong city. In Cologne, everyone drinks Kölsch, a blond beer served in a tall, cylindric glass, called *Stange*, or *stick* in English. In Düsseldorf, on the other hand, everyone drinks Altbier, a copper-colored beer served in any glass available. If one would order a Kölsch in Düsseldorf, or an Altbier in Cologne, one might make it to the 8 o'clock news, watching from a nearby ER, recovering from the repercussions.

I took the Autobahn, of course, and even though it is true that you can drive as fast as possible on it, it was, as usual, clogged with too much traffic to drive fast at all.

Three hours later, I arrived at my parents' doorstep. My mom, Uta, opened the door. Her pixie haircut was as short as ever. Maybe she had just been to the salon, but as always, her hair had stayed naturally white. I only knew her with white hair. Her hair had turned from brown to white when she was in her mid-twenties, and she had never colored it. No hair color, no nail polish, no makeup, just my beautiful mom.

"Inka!" she yelled, clutching my arm and hugging me awkwardly with the other while bending down. She pulled me inside and called for my dad to come, quickly, before I could even say hello.

My dad, Wilhelm, came around the corner shortly after, taking the place of my mom to hug me. He, too, had to bend down a little, as all the members of my family are tall except me. His short brown curls tickled my ear, and his glasses sat askew on his nose.

"What a wonderful surprise," he said, and I followed him inside.

Finally. Home.

My mom immediately ran to start the coffee machine, and my dad placed the obligatory sewing kit tin filled with cookies onto the huge wooden table in their sunroom, where we could take in the big forest that surrounded their property. Once we were all settled, steaming cups of coffee in front of us, cookie in hand, I dropped the bomb. I told them I was dying, once again.

"What do you mean?" my mom asked, her brows furrowed, not quite sure what I was getting at. "Did your doctor say anything? Did he say something at your last checkup appointment that you didn't tell us about? Is it the CF or is it something else?"

"Geez, Mom." I rolled my eyes. One of the biggest fears of my mom: being kept in the dark when it was about my health. Not being asked to dig through the vast medical knowledge she had acquired over the years and being allowed to help. "*My doctor* didn't say I was dying. *I* say I'm dying. I can feel my liver failing. The ascites is bad, I don't eat enough, I feel like shit most of the time, and today at university I just realized, there's only one thing left to do: get a new liver. Get listed for an organ transplant."

My mom dropped her cookie and had to dive under the table to retrieve it, while my dad and I just looked at each other across the table. He reached out his hand, and I placed mine into his for a short moment of comfort.

When my mom resurfaced with her cookie in hand, she did so with a curd nod, a set jaw, and a decisive chew when the cookie finally found its destination. She digested the cookie and the news. Like my dad, bad news didn't paralyze her.

Bad news, since I could remember, was always handled the same way: It is what it is, now we have to deal with it. And that day was no different. Whatever devastation my parents felt, they didn't broadcast it. Instead, plans were made. First, I had to meet the right doctors to confirm my diagnosis. We had to choose the right hospital, call them, make an appointment, gather information ourselves. My mom was in her element. This is what she did best: rolling up her sleeves and getting to it. My dad's task was to find all the phone numbers she'd need to get the ball rolling. Everyone knew what they had to do; after all, they had more than two decades of experience with this.

I never met my brother. Life didn't give me the chance to. Malte was born on a cold Saturday morning, December 11, 1976. Born prematurely, after a bumpy pregnancy. My mom had been on bed rest for months to save him, to save their first and only son, but it didn't help. He only lived for twenty-four hours.

No one knew why he died. Doctors and friends said it was simply bad luck, and my parents were more than willing to believe that too. Just bad luck. There was no reason why they couldn't try again. They had always wanted multiple children, at least two, maybe even three, and they kept holding on to that dream. And then, two and a half years later, I was born. After a normal pregnancy, being full-term, I also entered the world on a cold Saturday morning. Only difference, everything seemed perfect this time around, until again, twenty-four hours later, my parents received another death sentence. I was diagnosed with CF, and the doctors were sure I wouldn't make it past the age of four.

On a hunch, presumptions were phrased that Malte had been a victim of CF as well. Suddenly it wasn't bad luck anymore that had claimed him. It had been a genetic disorder, the same I was cursed with. A heartless nurse advised my mother to "better not bring any more children into this world," and that was it. Nobody knew much about cystic fibrosis back then. My parents were given a few recommendations, what to look out for, what to feed me, but how to keep me alive . . . they had to figure that out by themselves.

My mom immediately rolled up her sleeves and tried every therapy on me that was out there. She was determined to keep me alive and at the same time terrified to leave anything unused and be the reason for my dying even sooner. But after only three months of running from one therapy appointment to the next, always fearing she wasn't doing enough to keep her baby alive, she was burned out.

An emergency meeting with close friends was held and, on that evening, sitting around our corner kitchen table, drinking wine, eating snacks, my parents realized what they were doing wrong: It wasn't enough to run from one therapy appointment to the next—they also had to find the courage to let me live. They had to find the courage to do the necessary amount of therapy *and* grant me the freedom to live life for the rest of the day. And they did.

I still had a lot of therapy growing up. Nebulizer treatments, autogenic drainage (a special breathing technique to free my airways of phlegm), intravenous antibiotic therapies, swallowing tons of medications in the form of pills, physiotherapy, and lots of exercising, mostly running.

It was my dad who came up with the idea of running. After reading multiple articles about the benefits of antibiotic therapy in CF patients, he asked himself a crucial question: "What does it help my daughter to kill all the bacteria in her lungs but not take care of the thick phlegm that's clogging her airways?"

And just like that, the therapy of running was born.

From that moment on, we ran miles and miles, almost every day, to force the phlegm out of my lungs. I ran when I felt good, and I especially ran when I felt bad. I ran with a fever, I ran when the coughing was bad. If I got a nosebleed or had to throw up, I'd push myself to run the next hundred yards.

It was tough. Often, I got into arguments with my dad because I didn't want to run another mile, while he forced me to run another one out of fear he wasn't doing enough to keep me alive. When I got really angry with him, I left him behind and ran faster to come home ten minutes before him, telling my mom what an idiot he was and locking myself in my room. When my dad came home, he often had tears in his eyes. It wasn't easy for me to always take care of my health, but it also wasn't easy for my parents to fight me when all they wanted was to keep me breathing.

With running and all the other therapies, I spent about two hours every day to stay alive, but the rest of the time I spent living. Living a life as normal as possible. I went to kindergarten, all the way up to high school. I had sleepovers with my friends, staying awake all night hunched over a Ouija board, going shopping, attending concerts. When I was older, I went to clubs and talked about boys, fashion, and the newest album from Nirvana. I did it all. My life had been a full one so far, and there was no way my parents would let it end at the age of twenty-two. They had been here before and knew what to do.

The next morning, before even having a cup of tea, my mom was already on the phone, organizing, taking care of the logistics. The night before, my dad had done some research on which clinic would be the right one for me, providing my mom with their phone number. Only one night's sleep later, she was already talking with the clinic my dad had chosen for me, the Hannover Medical School.

Hannover is a rather ugly city in Northern Germany, but back in 2001, it was *the* location for an organ transplant. Today, every bigger city in Germany performs organ transplants day in and day out, but in 2001, Hannover was leading when it came to transplant surgery and CF care. So, that's where my mom and I would go. On August 7, a little over two weeks from now, we would drive to Hannover and talk to doctors about a potential liver transplant. The ball was rolling, and there was no way to stop it. Once my parents were on the journey to save my life, there was nothing else I could do but ride along.

While my mom scribbled everything down into her calendar with sharp, rigid movements of her pen, my dad gave me a long and heartfelt hug. While my mom found comfort in getting busy, rushing five steps ahead in order to know what might be waiting for us in the future, my dad and I found comfort in the moment. Standing there, holding each other, embracing the now, because who knew how long we would still have each other.

2

The Blue Envelope

Staying with your parents when you're twenty-two years old and have already experienced the freedom of living alone isn't easy. But on the other hand, who doesn't like to be pampered once in a while? I sure did, and I made the most of it. I stayed for more than a week at my parents' house and enjoyed the daily routine they had. My parents were riding to the slow current of retired life, which I needed so much right now. It felt wonderful to start each morning with the kind of breakfast you only get at your parents': fresh buns, eggs, cheese, and sliced turkey, some jam, and coffee—complete with the rustling of my dad's newspaper. After breakfast, my mom and I would take a walk with the dog through the forest behind their house. It's a huge forest, covered by a network of narrow hiking trails that lead you all the way to the Netherlands. You could cross the border multiple times on a hike without even noticing, if it weren't for the signs suddenly switching to Dutch.

When we'd come back from our walks, it was time for lunch. Not a big lunch—most of the time, only a sandwich or the leftovers from last night's dinner. In the afternoon, we'd run some errands, play card games, read a book, drink another cup of coffee, chill. Every evening, my dad would cook dinner, always something I especially liked, and we'd wrap up the day with watching TV. The next morning, the same. I loved it. It felt like floating in a bubble without upcoming doctor visits or life-changing decisions to make. I felt like a child again. Everything was taken care of for me. I didn't have to worry, I didn't have to think of anything—not even university. Without saying it out loud, without intentionally coming to that decision, I had dropped out of university. There was no reason for me to sit through lectures when I didn't know if I'd live or not. Right now, I only had to live from one meal to another, sleep, and repeat. And I did. For nine days straight, until reality snuck up on me again.

It was a Wednesday, and my dad had to pick up car parts for his old Mercedes from a shop about an hour away. My mom had a routine doctor's appointment that left me home alone in the afternoon. At first, I wanted to take another walk with Fenja but quickly decided against it when I realized how hot it had gotten. I considered calling my best and longest friend Silke from high school. I hadn't told anyone about my health concerns, but I just couldn't get myself to dial her number. Telling my friends would ultimately burst the bubble I was living in, would make reality real again; how I wasn't just on vacation but living on a countdown. I wasn't ready for that yet. I needed a little more time before I could face the fear of my friends *and* my own. Just a little more time.

I turned on the TV and switched through all the channels, but there was nothing on worth watching. Remember, this was 2001. No Netflix, no Hulu, no streaming. I also didn't feel like reading, which left me with only one thing to do: go through the two boxes my dad had left for me in his office. According to him, they were filled with old stuff I had left behind when I had moved out, and he wanted me to look through them, decide what was worth saving, what could be thrown away, and mostly, what I was willing to take back to my apartment and not have him store any longer.

The boxes were not huge, maybe the size of two hand luggage trollies, and not heavy either. I was able to drag them both to the middle of the room. I sat down beside them, right on the old Persian carpet that covered most of the floor. It was a relic from the time my dad had run his own home textiles store, and it still reminded me with a smile of that time when I was allowed to jump from one pile of carpets to the next at his store, like no other kid was allowed to. I wondered if my dad had similar memories, good ones hopefully, of why the carpet was now part of his office. He had always been a collector; the white IKEA shelves covering every wall were filled with antique books, vintage car models, and boxes filled with articles about cars, mostly; some of them he had cut out of magazines when he was still a boy. I guess there was a reason for the two boxes in front of me. With warmth spreading through my body, I opened the first one.

I don't know what I had expected, maybe some books, old girly magazines, memorabilia from my childhood, but definitely not my former diaries. What were they doing here? Why weren't they at my apartment? Locked up behind impenetrable doors where no one would ever find them?

Hesitant, as if they contained biohazardous material, I took them all out and placed them on the carpet around me. There were ten altogether, and none of them had the flimsy lock they had originally come with. They were all readily available for anyone's eyes. *Verdammt.* Damn.

I picked one up and flipped through it. Page after page filled with endless, intimate details of teenage life. A boring teenage life, I knew that much. Being chronically ill, way too skinny, underdeveloped, and constantly coughing in a way that made everyone think I might die didn't make me very popular, especially not with the boys. Everything written in these diaries was solely based on wishful thinking, daydreaming, or the experience of my friends.

I threw the diary back into the pile and grabbed one of those huge, thirty-gallon trash bags from the kitchen. The black ones, the heavy-duty ones, the ones that were made to keep biohazardous material sealed from the world until incinerated. I wanted to throw all of them away; if I weren't German, I might have considered my own book burning, but eventually, I couldn't do it.

First, I was terrified of what would happen if anyone found them, took them out of my parents' trash can, and read them. What if a strong wind blew them out of the trash can, spread them throughout the neighborhood, and every neighbor would get to read one of them? Ridiculous, I know, but still. And second, lame or not, they were proof that I had lived these angst-dominated teenage years, that I had been here, at least that.

I put them all to the side, on the pile I wanted to take back to my place. Keep them safe till the end of time.

There was nothing else inside the first box besides the diaries. The second box, though, turned out to be more interesting to look at and read through. It contained a huge pile of stories I had once written, many of them still on my dad's electric typewriter—poems, essays from school, drawings, and magazine articles I had collected over the years. Yes, I was definitely my father's daughter. I read through all of them. My own stories landed on the "take back to my place" pile; most of the articles, paintings, and school essays in the black, heavy-duty trash bag.

After an hour of work, I was done. I brought the trash out to the recycle bin, put one of the empty boxes on the side for my dad to use for something else, and used the other one to place all the things in it I had decided to take back to my place. But a blue envelope slipped out of a diary and landed on the floor. I didn't have to pick it up or even open it—I knew immediately what it contained. A letter that should have been in a safe place, not stored in between the pages of one of my disposable diaries. A letter I had read many times growing up. A letter from my dead uncle.

Carefully, as if it could dissolve into dust, I pulled the letter out of its blue envelope, unfolded it, and read:

> March 8, 1979
>
> Dear Inka,
>
> or
>
> Dear Ole (in case you will be born a boy),
>
> For the longest time I couldn't make up my mind—should I write to you or should I not. And if I write, how to begin? What to say? How to address you? The one person I will never get to know.
>
> I'm sure I don't have to explain myself, you will know my story by now, when you are old enough to read these immature lines, but I still need to spell it out, even if it's just for myself: We will never get to know each other, probably never even meet each other, because I'm dying. The big C. Lymphoma.
>
> I'm at the hospital right now, your dad is on his way to pick me up to bring me home to my wife, for me to hug her one last time, to say my final goodbyes, but I made my peace with it. It might sound weird,

but truly, I can consider myself lucky. The lymphoma grew much slower than doctors had predicted. When diagnosed, they gave me one year to live—that was nine years ago. But still, even nine years flew by in the blink of an eye. I held on as tight as I could, and still, time ran through my fingers like pudding through a sieve.

But what am I talking about? I'm not writing to scare or depress you. I'm writing to simply say Hello, to introduce myself, and to wish you all the best for your upcoming life. It feels to me like we will switch places. I will go and you will take over. Maybe that's why I'm writing to you today because you will take over the baton of life from me, carry it on, make it count and worthy. I know you will.

My dear, live your life! Enjoy your life! Laugh, adventure, and savor the ride. Because even if you live up to an old age, will be able to look back onto many, many years, it will still be a short one. And the most amazing one you will ever experience! You will see.

I can't wait to hear all about your adventures when you will sit beside me on cloud nine, many, many years from now, and tell me all about it.
I will always keep an eye on you, I will always be your uncle, always think of you.

Ingo

Two days after Ingo had written that letter, he was dead. And only one week later, I was born. On March 17, 1979. We truly did switch places. He left and gave the baton of life to me so I could start my own adventures.

I refolded the letter, placed it back inside the blue envelope, and put it on top of the "take back to my place" box. Then I just sat there, drew my legs and arms close to my body, and stared out my dad's office window. I watched the huge, dark green Rhododendron that surrounded their garden move slightly in the summer breeze. I felt a common sadness rushing in. The same sadness I always felt when I read Ingo's letter. He had wished so much for me. He had been sure I would live the life he never had—a healthy life. A life without hospital stays, without needles being poked into veins, without handfuls of medications that had to be swallowed every day, and most of all, a life without an early death. And here I was, twenty-two years old, sixteen years younger than Ingo had been when he died, and already having death breathing down my neck. What would Ingo say if I'd come to sit beside him on cloud nine after having lived for only twenty-two years? He'd be disappointed; same as I.

I heard my dog jump from the sofa in the living room, saw her running past my dad's office to the front door, where my mom was just getting out of her car. She was back from her doctor's appointment. Time for me to snap out of any sadness I was feeling, put back on a happy face, and not dwell any longer over what Ingo had wished for my life. It didn't matter. Or maybe I didn't want it to matter.

Before I went to open the front door for my mom, I slid the letter back in between the pages of the diary it had fallen out of. It wasn't that I didn't want my mom to see the letter. She knew the letter. She had read it probably as many times as I. Ingo had been her brother, after all, but that day, I didn't feel like bringing him up again. The letter had been addressed to me, not to my whole family, and that's where it would be from now on—with me. Same as my worry that I might meet Ingo much sooner than anticipated.

3

Just a Straw

Enough was enough.

It was time for me to drive back home. Back to Oldenburg. I needed time for myself. My parents' hovering was starting to annoy me. Not that their caretaking had morphed into coddling, but I had to go back to being an adult, back to taking care of things by myself. I needed to find some solitude to prepare myself for the upcoming hospital visit on August 7 too. The day I would find out how my life would continue, if at all. In addition, I also had to find ideas of how to fill my university-free days from now on, and, this was most crucial, I had to tell my friends about my health concerns. They deserved to know. I hated it, and a small part of me wished I could just do what I always did when I received bad news: keep them to myself until I found a solution.

But I knew, this time I had to allow my friends to worry alongside me. I couldn't just send them a postcard after my liver transplant, telling them I was fine, or worst-case scenario, have my parents send them an invitation to my funeral. I knew they wanted to worry alongside me, and that's why I sent all of them the same email:

June 15, 2001

Hello everyone,

I'm writing to all of you today to share some not-so-great news with you. Right now, I'm not feeling very well. My liver has worsened a lot lately. I have water in my abdomen, water in my legs, I'm short of breath because the swollen belly presses against my lungs, and my back hurts, because I also have to carry that water-filled belly of mine around. It might sound a little whiny, but unfortunately this is reality. Because of it all, I will talk with my doctors about a possible liver transplant.

The transplant, the risks involved—I try to deal with it. It's not that I have any other option. I will tell you guys more once I have talked to my doctors.

My psychology degree is canceled right now. I can't concentrate on psychology with what's going on anyway. Hopefully I will be able to pick it back up later, once I'm better again.

This is all. I don't have more to tell you, except I won't give up that easily!

Best,
Inka

August 7 was a rather cold and cloudy Tuesday in Northern Germany—weather as usual. I met up with my mom in the parking lot of the Hannover Medical School. We had decided that everyone drive by themselves; it was easier that way since we were coming from different areas of Germany. Rows of gray, rectangular windows greeted us while we looked up to them, praying to find what we were searching for behind these walls. Together, we walked toward the entrance.

The Hannover Medical School was built in the 1960s and radiates, as every building from the '60s, depression and helplessness rather than hope and medical miracles. I wanted to race my mom to the doctor's office to speed up time, to be done with it and out of there; at the same time, I wanted to turn around, run back to my car, and flee. What if I wouldn't find what I was looking for behind these walls? What if there was no medical miracle waiting for me here? No procedure known of that could lengthen my life.

My mom grabbed my hand, squeezed it reassuringly as if she could hear my thoughts, and with an empty feeling in the pit of my stomach, we stepped inside the hospital through its sliding doors. Our first appointment was with the cystic fibrosis department. First, the CF doctors would take a look at me and only then, if declared needed, would we go and see the liver transplant doctors. One doctor at a time.

We asked the way-too-happy lady at the front desk where to go. I wish I would've been allowed to smack the smile off her face. We took one of six available elevators she pointed to up to the CF department floor, checked in there with another overly friendly but distant-looking lady, and then sat in the waiting room, waiting to be called in for our appointment, just like everyone else.

At first, I was busy filling out a million papers to answer any question imaginable about my former life as a CF patient, but as it always does, boredom found me.

"We will sit here forever," my mom whispered in my ear, clenching her teeth, as if I didn't know that already. Nobody had been called since we arrived. Nothing had moved in the waiting room apart from tapped feet and greasy magazine pages printed during the last century.

"Why would Hannover be any different from other hospitals?" I whispered back and reached for my book.

Unimaginably long wait times in hospitals were nothing new. Waiting for two hours for an X-ray was normal, and the reason for it? Germany's universal multi-payer health care system.

Health insurance is mandatory in Germany, which means everyone is insured by a statutory health insurance. Everyone gets care, everyone has to pay a deductible according to their income, and everyone gets the same care unless one is fortunate enough to also have private health insurance. Apart from the deductible, every procedure is free of cost, as long as it's approved by the insurance.

In many ways, this was amazing, especially for someone like me. If I did need a liver transplant, I'd get approval from my insurance, pay my deductible, and that was it. Everything else would be covered by my insurance.

The downside of it was overloaded hospitals, long waiting times (sometimes people had to wait weeks before they could get an MRI), and doctors who were anything but customer oriented.

In America, doctors must listen to your concerns, your questions, and your wishes, because if they don't, you'll give that doctor a bad rating and go somewhere else. In Germany, however, you often got the feeling the doctor was primarily working for the insurance that pays their income, but not so much for you, the patient. Doctor visits in Germany often feel rushed; the doctor suggests what should be done next but doesn't have the time to discuss the decision with you, because they need to run to the next patient. A weird opposite to the long waiting times you have to spend up front to actually see a doctor.

I spent my waiting time reading; after all, I was an experienced hospital visitor and never came without a book handy, but after a bit, even I got tired of reading and started to examine the other patients who were waiting with us. There was simply nothing else to look at inside our waiting room. White walls, worn chairs, a coffee machine that hadn't been cleaned since the beginning of time, said greasy magazines, two askew picture frames with mountain views in them—nothing you could find anywhere near Northern Germany—and the other four patients, all of whom looked way sicker than I felt.

One of them, a girl maybe a few years younger than me, had an oxygen tube stuck under her nose. Her mom was asking her all the time if she needed anything, which she declined constantly without even looking up. They both looked stressed. Stressed and exhausted from too many hospital visits and too-long hours of waiting. Who could blame them.

Another girl, this one probably in her early teens, had come accompanied by an IV pole and a huge bag of liquid dangling above that dripped slowly into her vein. She also had someone with her, probably her mom too. All of us had adult company, including the guy about my age who was sitting furthest from us, coughing his lungs out every few minutes.

The third girl, sitting beside me, was wearing a mask over her face. I was sure she was already transplanted—lungs, though, not liver. This was 2001, so the only people wearing masks were those who had a compromised immune system due to an organ transplant. I considered for a moment to ask her if I had guessed right: *Was* she a lung transplant recipient? I wanted to know if the transplant had given her a new life, or if she was still struggling with shortness of breath and all the other CF-related stuff people like us struggled with. But I chickened out. I didn't want to intrude . . . and anyway, I wasn't there for a lung transplant. I was there because of my liver. We were fighting in different leagues and mine, I was sure of it, was the one with a higher chance of success. I only needed a new liver. I would be up and running again in no time. Piece of cake. I almost felt invincible, especially after comparing myself to the patients around me.

I wasn't out of breath like the others, true, but I didn't have oxygen stuck under my nose or an IV in my arm. I might have had the most swollen belly, but I was sure none of the other patients were still walking their dog, if they even had one. I was in great shape. I only needed a new liver, no big deal. My lungs were great, I felt great, everything would be great.

Great, great, great.

Relaxed and reassured, I grabbed one of the old and greasy magazines from the empty chair beside me and passed the remaining time reading about the hottest summer fashion trends of five years ago.

When my name was called, ninety minutes past our arrival, I first had to do a pulmonary function test. Nothing I hadn't done countless times before. My mom waited outside in the hall while I did my breathing test.

"FEV1 is at 950ml," the technician said and handed me a printout of my results.

I looked at it and was a bit surprised. The FEV1 measured the volume of air someone could press out of their lungs in one second. Being able to breathe out 950ml of air in one second was not much. Not much at all. If I'd been healthy, the amount should have been around 3,500ml. The difference spoke for itself.

After the pulmonary function test, my mom and I were seated inside one of the examination rooms, another depressingly white room with nothing but three chairs and white cabinets covering the windowless walls. We were asked to wait, once again.

"You wanna see the printout from the pulmonary function test?" I asked Mom the moment the door closed behind the nurse.

"Sure," my mom said with a cheer, not picking up on my hollow expression and hanging head.

I handed her the printout, and it took her a moment to find the FEV1, but when she did, she reacted like I had.

"Only 950ml? Is that even accurate?" Her body seemed to shrink, while she let out a hard sigh and closed her eyes.

"I'm afraid so." I searched for something to look at beside my caved-in mom, but there was nothing. One white cabinet beside another, nothing to stop my inner recycling of bleak thoughts: *This is it. I'm fucked. My liver is bad, my lungs are too. That's it. That's the end.*

Apparently, it was one thing to know you weren't that healthy anymore, but a completely different thing to see it printed in black and white.

"This looks bad, doesn't it?" I avoided eye contact to make it less real somehow. How was it possible that only thirty minutes ago I had felt oh-so healthy, comparing myself to the girl with oxygen under her nose. And now it seemed as if I was only one step away from standing in her shoes.

My mom nodded. She looked again at the printout, folded it up, put it in her purse, and then waved it all off with a sharp gesture of her arm.

"First, we need to see what the doctors will say," she said. "That's what we came here for. A professional opinion, not a single printout to freak out over. Let's just wait and see. We can still freak out later."

With that, she crossed her arms over her chest and clenched her teeth, as if denial would put off what was coming at us.

"But what do we do if my lungs are failing too?" I couldn't just sit there, cross my arms, and not freak out. My heart was racing, my chest felt tight and painful, as if it had decided to join my lungs and liver in being completely useless.

"You are still breathing, right?" my mom asked.

I nodded. "Kinda."

"The pulmonary function test only shows you a snapshot." My mom obviously wasn't ready yet to let go of wishful thinking and face reality. "It's not proof for anything," she continued. "We first have to wait for what the doctors have to say. And if they say the lungs look bad too, then we do whatever it takes to improve them. But first we have to wait for their professional opinion. First, we have to wait."

I opened my mouth, and then I closed it again, not knowing what to say. My mom was, as always, already a few steps ahead of me. Ready for a game plan, put together by the glorious physicians of the Hannover Medical School. I wasn't there yet at all.

How could my lungs be failing me too? How was that even possible when I was still walking my dog every day—long walks, walks that took over an hour? I was still doing everything at home, like any healthy person did. Laundry, grocery shopping, cooking, cleaning, hanging out with my roommate, sometimes even going out to have a coffee somewhere. None of this made sense. A failing liver *and* failing lungs? I wish I had the belief of my mom that there was a cure for it, but I couldn't.

We didn't have to wait for long for our doctor to come see us. Thank God, because my doomsday thoughts were driving me crazy. If there was no cure for a failing liver and failing lungs, I would be dead. Figuratively and literally speaking. Something I wasn't equipped to hear. Not. At. All. Just thinking about it, I felt like passing out while having a heart attack. There had to be something that could be done. Anything. I didn't care what it was—I just needed a straw to hold on to. Just a straw, nothing more.

My doctor didn't waste much time going over the test results. She knew I was in deep shit, and she knew we knew just as much. She asked a few benign questions, how I felt, how I would describe the decline of my health, what had caused me to believe I needed a liver transplant, until she mentioned the bad performance of my lungs.

"Inka," she said matter-of-factly, "your lungs, even though it seems like it, aren't bad enough to consider a lung transplant."

My mom and I exchanged a quick look and exhaled in unison. No lung transplant—so far so good.

"But . . ." she continued with a firm voice, looking straight into my eyes, "a liver transplant by itself won't save you either."

"What?" My mom gasped, then shook her head with decisiveness. "I don't understand. That doesn't make sense."

I turned my head to look at her, then wanted to scream at her, "What don't you understand? I don't need new lungs, and a liver won't save me. I'm fucking done." But I just sat there, shrinking into my chair, feeling cold and numb. There was no miracle waiting for me at the Hannover Medical School. No glorious doctors who would do everything in their power to save my life, because there was nothing out there that *could* save my life.

I suddenly wanted to stand up and leave. I didn't want to talk anymore, I didn't want to hear anything anymore, I only wanted to go home, crawl into my bed, and cry. I grabbed my bag, ready to stand up, when my doctor said:

"The only chance Inka has is a combined lung *and* liver transplant. Not liver, not lungs, but both organs together."

"A what? A lung and liver transplant?" I asked, feeling as if I had missed the last five minutes of the show and now had no idea what we were talking about. "Didn't you just say a liver transplant won't save my life, and now you're talking about a liver *and* a lung transplant. That doesn't make sense at all." I felt hot. My mind raced to find answers. What the hell was going on here? Had my doctor lost her mind? Lungs and liver? I looked at my mom, hoping she would come up with an interruption or some kind of delay to end this madness, but she just sat there with a blank expression on her face.

"Let me explain the reasons behind a combined lung and liver transplant," my doctor said into the silence of the room, and she did. She explained how once I'd receive a liver transplant, I'd have to take medications that would suppress my immune system. These medications were necessary to prevent my body from rejecting the new liver like it would, say, a virus. But a suppressed immune system would also allow the bacteria and fungi in my lungs to multiply and multiply (like every CF patient, I had plenty of bacteria and fungi). My now-still-functional lungs would be destroyed within a short period, being overrun by bacteria and fungi, and I'd find myself again on the organ transplant waiting list—only this time for a set of new lungs. The only way to prevent this from happening was to transplant both organs right away, together.

A double lung and liver transplant.

Fuck!

4

A Chance

Now it all made sense. All this madness finally clicked: this was exactly the miracle I had hoped for. A single liver wouldn't save me, but a liver combined with new lungs *might*. Not everything was lost yet. Not yet.

My mom was as shell-shocked as I was but quickly found comfort in planning the next steps. What had to be done to get me on the waiting list? Which doctors did we have to see next? Who would contact my health insurance and make them understand that they had to pay for all of this? I, on the other hand, found comfort in being stubborn.

Not just a new liver, but also new lungs? *Pff*, no problem, I could do that. I might have been wrong thinking I was still the healthiest of all, but I would be the healthiest of all double lung and liver transplant recipients. Done. I would show them, all of them, whoever they might have been, that I wasn't done living. I'd just refuse to die, refuse to be sick, and go from there.

I was able to keep my fear under control while my mom kept talking to my doctor. Thank God I had no idea of how rare my kind of combined transplant truly was. I had no idea how low my chances of surviving it were. I didn't know how little experience anyone had with this kind of procedure. I only knew there was still a chance for me to survive, and that's all I needed. A chance. I didn't need a guarantee. I didn't need great numbers or a high success rate. I only needed a chance, and a chance I got. The rest I would concur with being stubborn and being angry. Anything was better than feeling defeated or scared.

During the years of 2000 and 2001, there had been five double lung and liver transplants in Europe. Three of these five transplants had taken place in Hannover and were described as a success when the patient had survived the first-year post-transplant, which the last two double lung and liver transplant recipients of Hannover hadn't. The USA, as a comparison, had performed two double lung and liver transplants during the years of 2000 and 2001.

The combination of lungs and liver was and still is a rare one, and one that is often not blessed with much success. Up until today (November 1, 2022), there have been 163 double lung and liver transplants in the USA. Compared to that stand 48,096 lung transplants.

Our conversation with the CF doctor was short but not rushed. Or maybe my mom and I were still too dumbstruck to feel much of anything.

When we were done, once my mom had asked all the questions she could come up with, we were told to make a follow-up appointment, and then go over to see one of the liver transplant specialists. Even though my CF doctor had already decided on a lung transplant in combination with the needed liver, the liver specialists had to agree with this approach before any further steps were taken.

The overly friendly but distant lady at the check-in scheduled our follow-up appointment and then explained to my mom how we'd get to the liver transplant department. It was on the other side of campus, in a different building, miles away from what it felt to me.

“I’m tired,” I said with slumped shoulders while we were waiting for the elevator to take us down again to ground level. “And hungry too. And grumpy.”

My mom smiled. She looked tired as well, like she had to carry every word the doctor just told us on her back, but not as defeated as I felt. “Yeah, I can tell,” she said. “How about we eat something downstairs before we continue. What do they call the place downstairs again?”

“The shopping street.” I rolled my eyes. “They make it sound like 6th Avenue. The shopping street,” I repeated louder than necessary and raised my arms in glory. “For sure it’s just a lame kiosk with prewrapped sandwiches and drip coffee that’s been sitting on a hot plate since 1995.”

But I was wrong. The *shopping street* of the Hannover Medical School truly was a tiny 6th Avenue, minus the fancy. When you entered the hospital and didn’t take the elevators as we did when we arrived, you were basically there. On your right side you could find a hairdresser, a bookstore stocked with medical books as well as novels, a kiosk, yes, where you could buy snacks, candy, and magazines, and a café.

My mom and I stopped at the café, and we were positively surprised. Having spent a fair amount of my life in hospitals, I knew not to expect much when it came to food that was made, bought, and/or served inside any of them. But this café offered a reasonable selection of meals, drinks, and even cake. My stomach rumbled in anticipation.

“Are we going to sit down?” I asked my mom. The surroundings were rather nice. Inside the café were only a few tables, all of them occupied, but on the other side of the café was a huge window front looking out to the hospital’s garden. It wasn’t an English garden, but one could see green lawn, big trees, and a few maintained flower beds. From time to time, a visitor and patient strolled by or sat on one of the benches outside. It was nice.

"We could sit over there." I pointed to rows of chairs and a few couches that were placed alongside the garden windows, which looked as if they had been stolen from an IRS office, but I didn't care. I needed a break. A short moment of normality, eating lunch, watching people walking down Hannover's 6th Avenue, while drinking a huge cup of coffee and not thinking of anything else. Snuggles for the soul.

I ordered toast Hawaii—like a Hawaiian pizza, but just on toast—and my mom got herself a cheese sandwich. And for both of us, the biggest café au lait they had to offer, the early version of the later coffee latte.

We sat down on one of the couches, balancing our plates on our knees, surrounded by plastic palm trees, sterile hospital air, and shoes squeaking over linoleum. My mom called my dad to tell him what we had learned so far. I peeled the pineapple off my toast because it was not what I had expected. I watched doctors, nurses, patients, and visitors pass by. I tried not to think of anything. I felt empty. Empty and emotionally exhausted. I could hear my mom beside me, telling my dad the next steps we had to take, seeing the liver doctors, how to get on the transplant waiting list. As usual, she was ten steps ahead.

I couldn't help but wonder what my dad was thinking. Probably he was still stuck on the first thing my mom had told him. How we were not facing a sole liver transplant anymore, but also lungs. I knew I was still stuck on this one, still trying to digest it, to wrap my head around it. I had so many questions rushing through my head. I didn't know what to do next other than to follow the tasks my mom was already piling up in her planner.

"Next, we'll go see the liver transplant doctors," I heard her say to my dad. I wondered if he felt as lost in the flood of new information as I did.

I sighed, stood up to throw my pineapple in the trash, and then reached out for my mom to hand me her empty plate as well so I could return them to the café.

When I came back, she was done talking.

"Okay. Let's do this." She stood up and brushed crumbs off her jacket, ready to roll. "One more stop. Hopefully we won't have to wait too long to see one of the liver doctors. Hopefully we will be out of here by two p.m."

The second we stepped into the beautiful, light-flooded and flower-decorated waiting room of the liver department, I couldn't believe it either. I *knew* we wouldn't be out of there by 2:00 p.m. It was crowded. There were probably twenty other patients waiting to be seen, sitting on newly upholstered chairs, reading magazines from only two years ago, and now us as well.

Again, I filled out a whole booklet of forms, flipped through a set of not-so-old and greasy magazines, until finally, after another ninety minutes of waiting time, my name was called. Not by a nurse, but by one of the liver doctors himself.

He looked more like an accountant to me than a doctor. Ironed all over in sharp edges. While he waited for us to gather our things, he flipped through the paperwork I had just filled out, and the test results from earlier this morning. He nodded a few times, apparently in agreement with what the CF doctors were thinking, and then asked us to follow him to one of the examination rooms.

My mom and I shuffled after him through a busy narrow hall lined with doors to our right and left.

"It's full today," my doctor told us back over his shoulder as an excuse or an explanation for the crowding. He was about to open one of the doors for us when another white-coated doctor—this one older with graying thin hair and a bored look of too many years at this department—passed us in the hall and was stopped by my doctor in his tracks.

"Professor, may I have a moment?" my doctor asked, blocking the other one's path. "Could you please have a quick look at this patient of mine?" He pointed at me, handed over some of the documents he had been flipping through, and waited.

We all waited. Right there, in the middle of the hall. Nurses squeezed by, doctors, one patient—no privacy needed because no one cared. Everyone had their own health problems on their mind.

"Definitely," the professor said, as if there was nothing left to say. He handed the papers back to my doctor, took a quick glance at me, and clarified, "Yes, she definitely needs a liver transplant."

"Thank you," my doctor said, and that was it. We didn't get to see the examination room. I didn't get to know the name of the professor who had decided on my liver transplant by flipping through some pages in the hall. I wasn't asked any questions. I wasn't examined, and we weren't told why we had come at all since my presence was obviously unnecessary.

My doctor ushered us back to the front desk. We were asked to make a follow-up appointment to discuss further details, and then he vanished with a hasty "goodbye" to hopefully show the next patient the inside of an examination room.

"Um . . ." My mom waved after our doctor, who was already gone, trying to catch up with what had just happened.

"You need a follow-up appointment?" the receptionist behind the desk reminded her and gave my mom a nodding smile.

"Yes, I guess," my mom said while I decided to wait outside, behind the closed doors of the liver transplant department, trying to resurrect my stubbornness to avoid any other kind of feelings. I wanted to be angry, determined, pissed off that I had to deal with all of this. Anything but fear, doubt, and confusion about what was going on.

Just like that, it was decided: a liver *and* a lung transplant. Not that I had any doubt of what the liver experts would say, but being discarded like I had been, with only one glance of my test results before declaring my liver was indeed failing, was, even for German standards, considered disrespectful. I understood why the professor without a name or manners didn't need to hear my whole story to know I needed a transplant. I mean, even I knew. I also understood why he wasn't ready to listen to my concerns, my fears, or to be confronted with any kind of human emotions. He was a doctor, a doctor who took care of the largest solid organ inside the human body, a doctor who took care of the body's filtration system. Emotions? Not his concern, but still, they should have been. I was only twenty-two years old. I had just gotten the confirmation that my life was ending, would be ending, if I didn't get a transplant so huge, I hadn't even known it existed until a few hours ago. I was terrified, confused, and left alone with an obstacle so monumental, I didn't know how to go about it. When my mom found me outside, I collapsed in her arms and cried. It didn't take her long to join me.

On our way back to our cars, my mom called my dad again to give him the final update. He didn't say much, told her to give me a hug, to drive carefully, and that they would talk once she was back home.

When we reached our cars, my mom digging for her keys in her purse, I finally found my voice again.

"And what do we do now?" I asked.

She looked up from her purse. "What do you mean?"

"I mean, what do we do now?" I repeated with a hint of frustration. "Just drive home and then what? What's going to be the next thing we need to do to get this . . . shitshow started?"

My mom raised one eyebrow but didn't comment on my cussing. Instead, she let me know that our follow-up appointment with the liver people was in one week from now. "On August fourteenth," she said.

"Should we bring some folding chairs to sit in the hall while one of their professors talks to us, or will we actually get to see one of their examination rooms this time?"

My stubbornness and my anger were coming back, and I was glad they were. I didn't like falling apart, being consumed by fear. I preferred sarcasm and being insufferable. My mom, maybe not so much.

"I was told," my mom said, saying each word with deliberate calm, "that our next appointment will take about an hour. We will be able to ask all our questions, we will get all the information we need, and yes, I assume we will be allowed in one of their examination rooms and offered chairs this time."

She finally got her car keys out of her purse, unlocked the door, and looked at me, ready to say goodbye.

"I think next week we should also ask Tina to come join us. What do you think?"

"Like 'three pairs of ears hear more than two' kinda thing?" I asked.

She nodded. It was a great idea to bring my six-years-older sister along with us. Not only to ask potential medical questions, but also for additional emotional support. Which I was sure I'd need.

"I'll call her when I get home." I hugged my mom as tight as possible. One step at a time. We would get there, eventually.

When I got to my car, buckled in, and turned the key, the dashboard clock read 2:01 p.m. We had made it after all. Thanks to the lengthy three-minute conversation with the liver transplant professor.

5

Medical Miracle

When I got home from my hospital visit, I first brought my roommate Aria up to date. We sat in our kitchen, drinking coffee and talking about what was going to happen or what I believed was up ahead. Most of the time I knew as much as Aria, which was nothing, but talking helped both of us to digest the shock of it all.

After our coffees were finished, Aria went back to her normal afternoon activities, taking care of whatever she had to take care of for her business degree, and I finally called my sister on the landline. Calling a cell phone in 2001 was entirely restricted to emergencies—life-or-death emergencies—since it cost an arm and a leg to actually use your cell phone back then. And of course, my cordless landline phone wasn't charged, damn me.

I let the phone ring ten times before I hung up. Apparently, my sister wasn't home. If I wanted to talk to her, I had to call her cell.

I swiveled in my chair, outstretching the telephone cord, and tried to decide if the situation was critical enough to call my sister on her cell.

"Ah, fuck it." I dialed her number.

Tina picked up on the sixth ring, a little out of breath and obviously occupied.

"Hey," she said. "You are calling me on my cell? All okay? Are you back home?"

"Yeah, I'm home. All good, just wanted to give you all the news. Do you have a minute?"

I heard some shuffling, and something fell to the floor with a loud cladder, then my sister again.

"Yeah, give me a second. I'm in the stable right now, but I can finish later. One second."

My sister was a veterinarian, specializing in horses. She lived in the downstairs apartment of the stable's owners. She took care of all their horses, her own horse included, and otherwise drove around to other stables in the area to see additional clients. She truly lived in the countryside and had a life that was absolutely foreign to the rest of the family. Relatives of my grandfather had a farm somewhere in eastern Germany—cows and pigs—but none of us, including my grandfather, had ever spent a day working on a farm. But my sister loved it. Working outside, being surrounded by animals and their animal-loving owners, the dirt, the one million flies that landed on whatever food you dared to unwrap out there—my sister was happy where she was.

I could hear a bolt closing, a horse neighing, then Tina's heavy booted steps walking from the stable's boxes over to her apartment. A little more rustling, her boots being dumped onto the floor, and finally, she was back with me.

"Okay," she said through a big sigh, "want me to call you back on the landline? Dad will have a heart attack when he sees your phone bill."

"Yeah, that might be best. Will take a few minutes to bring you up to date."

We both hung up, and a few seconds later, my landline rang.

"Okay," my sister said after another rustling sound. She probably had to remove two loads of unfolded laundry from the sofa to be able to sit down. "I'm ready. Tell me everything. What did the doctors say?"

And I did. I told her everything.

She couldn't believe what I was telling her.

"Lungs and liver? Why?" she asked, same as my mom and I had asked a few hours earlier. I explained to her everything the doctors had explained to us, and I could imagine the shaking of her head as the magnitude of what was happening slowly sank in.

"This is crazy," she said, and I couldn't agree with her more, "but what are we doing now?"

Just like our mom, Tina was more fact-driven than emotional. She, too, found comfort in rolling up her sleeves and getting ready to deal with it. One of the reasons why I needed my sister for all of this: she and my mom would be the forces that would push me forward, push me to take the next step, push me to get transplanted and not just sit there, mourning what was already lost. When I ended my report, I asked if she would join Mom and me next week for my appointment in Hannover.

"Of course I'll join you." She let out a scoff. "Can't wait to finally use my folding chair for the first time sitting in the hall, listening to your professor."

And that was the other reason why I needed my sister by my side. She had the same morbid humor as me and our dad. The three of us always had an inappropriate comment on our lips, and we loved to share them.

When I was diagnosed with diabetes, I had to start poking myself multiple times a day to check my blood sugar. One of those times, I sat on the table opposite my dad, and when I poked myself, I exclaimed that it hurt. My dad glanced over, shrugged dismissively, and said: "Then you shouldn't poke yourself."

Then he went back to reading his newspaper.

This was exactly our way of dealing with the things that mattered so much they hurt deep inside. But instead of nourishing the hurt, we had decided to nourish our morbid humor instead.

And I loved it.

"I don't even have a folding chair," I said to my sister, going along with where she was taking the conversation.

"Too bad," my sister trilled. "Though I'm sure you can wait in the car. Your presence is not needed there anyway as it sounds."

We both laughed, made a few more inappropriate jokes about the liver transplant people, and then said goodbye. We would see each other in one week. I was happy. For the first time since I had heard the words *double lung and liver transplant*. All thanks to my sister. It always felt good talking to her, and it felt good to know that she assessed my situation the same as my doctors did. She understood immediately why I needed liver *and* lungs and agreed strongly with the decision Hannover had taken. Veterinary or otherwise, she came from a medical background and was able to understand and process everything that involved me and my situation in a different and more fact-oriented way. Not that I needed her reassurance that I was on the right path, but it still felt good to have it.

One week later, we all met in Hannover. My sister came together with my mom, and I in my own car. Just seeing the two of them, my sister as tall and athletic as my mom, her blond curls tied behind her neck, her attire as if she signed up for a two-week survival camp, I could already feel how this visit would be different. Not only that it was the three of us, but, stupid as it may sound, the sun was shining and made Hannover Medical School appear less depressing than last time. It was still the same ugly brick building, but in the sun, it radiated the medical miracle I was hoping for. Stepping with confident strides through the entrance's sliding door, I didn't feel uncertainty. I felt like I was destined to be there. Ready to get this transplant on its way.

We walked down the shopping street, heading for the other side of the building to get to the liver department. But Tina had a priority: coffee.

"But we just got here!" My mom sighed, threw up her arms, and quickly decided on a coffee au lait before she was left out.

"We will be late," I chimed in, but my sister wasn't having any of it. She has never been punctual. The world would wait for her, same as my doctors.

"Everything is better with coffee," she explained, "and we won't be late for our appointment. We will be late for our waiting time. I can live with that."

The liver department was well visited when we arrived, every one of us holding a steaming cup of coffee in hand, but by far not as crowded as it had been the last time. My sister immediately sat down, nursing her coffee, while my mom and I checked in.

"Okay," the receptionist said, "you are checked in, dear. It won't be long today. You should be called up pretty soon."

And the lady was right. We were called in after a little over thirty minutes of waiting time. It was just what the sun outside had promised. This time, our visit would be grand.

And it was.

After being called up, we were led into one of the examination rooms—no folding chairs needed—and two doctors came to see us.

One was a liver transplant doctor, and the other a lung transplant doctor. They gave us a wholesome introduction into the procedures of my transplant:

Both organs would be transplanted in one setting. First, the lungs, then the liver. The operation would take about eleven hours. After transplanting the lungs, they'd let me *rest* for two hours, while still under anesthesia, and only then start with the liver transplant. That was the common procedure.

The organs would both come from the same donor. The donor and I needed to have matching blood types and be approximately the same size, as the donor's lungs had to fit into my chest cavity. The liver could be cropped until fit, but the lungs only to a certain amount.

We asked a million questions. Medical ones (asked by my sister), organizational ones (asked by my mom), and the ones that were aiming at the future of how life would be after such an aggressive operation (asked by myself), but most of the answers I got were vague. There was no knowing how successful the transplant would be, the list of possible complications was endless, and to predict the future was something no one dared to even try. We had to wait and see. My transplant was not a guarantee for a healthy life afterward; it was barely a straw to hold on to . . . and hope not to slide off. Still, it was such a relief to get information and attention from not only one, but two doctors. With every answer we received, the whole undertaking felt more and more possible. There were certain procedures in place. Clear guidelines of what had to be done, when and how. This was not trial and error. This was an established surgical procedure, or at least that's what it felt like. We were in good hands. Hands that could make my medical miracle come true.

Our consultation had already exceeded the one hour it was scheduled for by more than thirty minutes, but before I was ready to say goodbye to the doctors, I had one more question. A question I was especially eager to get an answer to. A question I should have never asked.

The doctor leaned forward, as if ready to get up and leave.

"How long will it approximately take for me to get organs?" I blurted out. "How long do you think I have to wait for a new liver and new lungs?"

"Hard to say," the leaning-forward one said. "It can take a week; it can take months. But allow me to be completely blunt here: the right person has to die, including donor passport, for you to get transplanted. Everything needs to be a perfect match. It's not that easy, but . . ."

Now I leaned forward. I knew he was about to give me an estimate. Only an estimate, but still, I had to know. How long? How long?

"Yes?" I urged.

"But, based on statistics," he continued with slight hesitation, "we estimate a wait time of about three months."

"Okay." I leaned back, then looked at my mom and sister. Both had the same expression on their faces like I did. Three months was doable. Three months was great. I could definitely wait three months. Three months to get a new life.

Instantaneously, the number of three months burned itself into my prefrontal cortex. Three months, as in 91 days, 2,184 hours, or 131,040 minutes. And not a single second more.

Never have I ever believed anything a doctor told me with that much conviction. And never, ever had a doctor been so wrong.

A few things changed after our visit with the liver and lung transplant doctors. First, I got an oxygen concentrator. Only a few weeks after I had been sitting in the waiting room of the CF department, convinced I was the healthiest of all and wouldn't need oxygen for a very long time, life had shown me the middle finger. From now on, I had to sleep with a tube wrapped around my ears, stuck under my nose, to supply me with extra oxygen during the night.

"It'll help you have more energy during the day," one of the doctors had said, and even though I was absolutely against having an oxygen concentrator parked in my bedroom, he was right. The extra oxygen *did* help me during the day. It made me feel stronger, maybe even healthier.

I hated it.

I loved it.

Second, I got a prescription for a new medication, a diuretic, a so-called water pill. This pill would help me get rid of the water I had accumulated in my abdomen, the ascites, by simply telling my body to pee it out. That's why we called it the pee pill. Of course, my sister and I came up with the name. And the pee pill worked.

After only a few weeks, my belly was already less swollen. It wasn't pressing on my lungs anymore or tempting me to skip meals. I could button up my pants again and was more active again. The walks I did with my dog grew longer and longer, and I took care of multiple doctor visits I had to fulfill as preparation to be listed on the organ transplant waiting list. I couldn't wait to finally start counting off the three months of my waiting time. All the fear I had regarding the transplant was now accompanied by a small amount of hope.

I felt better since I got the extra oxygen during the night and since I was taking the pee pill. I felt like I had control over my body again. It wasn't only my body anymore dictating how my day was going; I was able to decide by myself what the upcoming day would hold for me. If I wanted to meet my friends in a café, I could. If I wanted to walk for another half an hour with my dog, no problem. Staying up a little longer to finish the movie I was watching, possible.

Of course, these were all baby steps. I wasn't suddenly cured and could climb Mount Everest on my lunch break if I wanted to, but to me these baby steps felt like I was able to climb mountains again. And if I was able to climb mountains, why not also move one of them and survive a lung and liver transplant?

I knew the surgery I was facing was enormous. As my doctors said, the list of possible complications was endless, but when you're twenty-two years old, complications, worst case scenarios, and death in particular don't seem to apply to you. I just couldn't imagine I would or even could die. Other people died, but not me. I was optimistic again, same as my dreams:

> September 2, 2001
>
> Last night I had an extraordinary dream. I was sitting with my uncle Ingo in a house, and we were chatting. Completely normal, as if we'd known each other forever. Around us was a little bit of commotion, I think someone was moving. And when I woke up, I knew one thing with absolute certainty: Ingo would, even though he was dead, watch over me during my waiting time and the transplant itself. No doubt at all. A nice thought, and it somehow calms me to know Ingo will be by my side. I'm sure he will do a great job!

Ingo again. I couldn't believe it. The box I had brought back to my place from my parents' home—the one with all my old diaries and

Ingo's letter in it—was still sitting in my living room, right beside my desk, untouched since I had parked it there.

It took me a second to find Ingo's letter. Another two to unfold it, and there it was again, right in front of me, spread out on my desk.

I looked at it for a while, tracing the lines of his writing with my eyes, how his N and U looked interchangeable, how every S had a little extra hock attached at the top, how everything was a mixture of block and cursive. He had written these words. He had moved his pen over this piece of paper, had held it in his hands, same as I was holding it now. It gave me chills. Like I was able to touch him by touching what he had touched.

There's a photo of my mom, my sister, Ingo's wife, and Ingo himself. They are all sitting on a sofa. Ingo is to the right, half of his body cut off by the picture's frame. To the left is his wife, right beside her my mom, my sister sitting on her lap. She was about five years old when the photo was taken.

Overall, it's not a good picture. Everyone is facing away from the camera, except Ingo, but he is half cut off. Like the person who took it didn't even bother to focus on anything, but I was still jealous of this particular moment. Because it showed how my sister had the privilege to get to meet Ingo. She had been in the same room with him. Had heard him laugh, talk, maybe she even sat on his lap for a while. She probably didn't remember—she wasn't even six when he died—but still, she had met him, and the picture was proof of it.

I wished I had a picture like that.

I put the letter back in its envelope, tucked it away in one of my desk drawers, and suddenly had an idea. A crazy idea, but who cared? Instead of writing in my diary, I would do something way better. I would write a letter to Ingo. An answer to his letter, a thank-you for visiting my dream. Because Ingo was someone I could be completely honest with. I could share all my fears with him without worrying about his own feelings. He would be my confidant. My connection to the other side.

I liked it, I liked it a lot.

I fished a simple piece of ruled paper out of my desk, grabbed a pen, and started to write:

> Dear Ingo,
>
> Finally, twenty-two years later, I'm writing back. But like you back then, I don't really know why I'm writing at all. I can't even leave these words behind for you, as there's no hope you'll read them someday. But still, or maybe because of it, I want to tell you what's going on in my life right now. Because you know as no one else how it feels to be faced with death. How it feels to waste your already limited lifetime in hospitals and have doctors torture you with needles and proclamations. You know, even though you didn't mention it in your letter, how shitty life can be. That it isn't just a gift to live, but a death sentence.
>
> Don't worry, I'm not as depressed as I may sound. I, too, am a fighter. If you want to grow old with cystic fibrosis, you must be. But honestly, I'm so fucking tired (excuse my language) of constantly fighting for my life. I don't want to be sick! I just want to study, live a boring life, grow old as you described in your letter. Instead, I'm facing an organ transplant.

Sometimes I ask myself: *What if I don't survive the transplant?* Or die while still waiting for it? Can life truly go on without me? What will my family do if I'm suddenly not there anymore? This question doesn't even seem real and still, I'm afraid of it.

On the other hand, my life isn't even worth living anymore. I don't live anymore, I vegetate. Alive or not, there isn't really a big difference. Which sums up to: I'm afraid to lose something that doesn't even exist anymore. I probably lost it already years ago, somewhere in between the last and the next hospital stay.

Ingo, why is life so complicated? Is it worth fighting for, even though I don't know if I'll get what I want? How does death feel in comparison to it? Is the seat beside you on cloud nine still free?

Sometimes I wish I could just sit down with you, dangle my legs, and not worry about life anymore. Sometimes . . .

I'll write to you again if there's something to share. —
Your not-as-depressed-as-she-may-sound-in-her-letter niece

A few days later, on a sunny Tuesday, a letter came in the mail. A letter from the Hannover Medical School:

> [...] *your medical situation was presented to our multidisciplinary liver and lung transplant committee. The decision made by the committee is that you are a candidate for a combined lung and liver transplant. Since 09/07/2001, you are actively listed on the organ transplant waiting list for a double lung and liver transplant* [...]

I jumped up from my chair, ran over to Aria, who was brooding over a marketing presentation, waved the letter in my hand, and screamed.

"I'm officially listed! I'm officially on the waiting list." I raised my arms over my head as if I had just won a marathon. "The three months of waiting time can start. By December, I will be transplanted. Yes. Yes! YES!"

Aria jumped up from her chair, and we did a little dance in her room, until I had to sit down because of a coughing fit that lasted for over a minute.

It sounded bad. As if I was about to suffocate, but Aria was no stranger to my coughing. She simply sat down beside me, took the letter out of my hands, read it for herself, and waited until my head wasn't tomato red anymore and I was able to breathe again.

"It's also a little bit scary, isn't it?" She absently twisted her hair, then pointed at the letter while rubbing her other hand in a constant stroke over her pant leg.

"Maybe," I said. "Why?"

"Because . . . I don't know." She shrugged, gave the letter back to me, and went to sit at her desk, looking out her window. "It's just scary," she said, still not looking at me. "How such a huge operation is only about three months away."

"Yeah." I got up. I was considering saying more, to actually say what we were both thinking, but decided against it, just like she had. We both felt it: with the news of a waiting time came the fear that I could be dead in three months. If I wouldn't survive my transplant, we would have only three months left together.

"Do you wanna see a movie tonight?" I asked, halfway out of her room. "Go to the movies together?"

She turned in her chair and finally looked at me.

"I'd love that. Yes." A huge smile lit up her face.

"How about this French movie called *Amélie*? You heard of it?"

She shook her head. "Is it a scary movie or more of a chick flick? I love chick flicks."

"It's not scary," I said. "But I mean, it's French. For sure it's weird."

"Never mind. Weird or not, let's just go and see it. Around six?"

I held up my thumb. Six was perfect. This was going to be a good day. I was officially listed, I had plans for tonight, life felt almost normal.

I went back to my room to call my parents and my sister. I had to share the great news of my being on the waiting list already for four days.

6

Certain Death

Oldenburg was known as *the* bicycle city in the north. Cyclists were everywhere: at the side of the road, in the middle of the road, on the sidewalk, parks, university campus. My physiotherapist's office was in the slow-paced, bicycle-infested Oldenburg. Though ten minutes from my house, it took longer to get to thanks to the constant yielding. But I was determined to show them what wonderful news I had received in the mail today.

The office itself was nothing that stood out in the common-place business area it was located in. A red brick one-story building of which one of the clear glass doors led to my physiotherapist, right beside a video library (an American Blockbuster) and a bicycle sale and repair shop, of course. Behind the glass door of my physiotherapist were two black treatment tables covered with a scratchy sheet of paper; right beside the gym corner were patients lifting weights and doing lunges, while I'd get stretched, pulled, and cranked back into shape. It was a painful experience every time. I never wanted to go but always did, only because the conversations with my therapist, the mom of a boy I went to elementary school with, kept me distracted enough not to run away.

The overall purpose for the painful treatment was to clear my airways, remove built-up mucus, improve lung function, increase mobility of the upper body, and loosen my shoulder muscles.

My shoulders were always tight and painful because I pulled them up all the time. Pulling up my shoulders somehow helped me to breathe and was also one of the reasons why most CF patients had bad posture. We all pulled up our shoulders. We all fought for each breath.

When I got in the car to drive to my physiotherapist, I turned on the radio and caught the end of the three o'clock news.

For the most part, they talked about the German secretary of defense. He did something that he wasn't supposed to do, I didn't really listen. Politics were not my problem right now.

Next, they had some news from New York. Apparently, a twin-engine plane had crashed into one of the Twin Towers of the World Trade Center. There was some smoke—nothing else was known yet.

It was probably a confused pilot, taking the wrong turn and then crashing into one of New York's skyscrapers. But I did wonder for a second how it was possible to hit a skyscraper by mistake. I mean, a skyscraper? If there was anything you could see from far away, it sure was a 110-story-high building.

I took a few more turns and arrived at my physiotherapy. Half an hour of pain waited for me. I parked my car in the half-empty parking lot, gathered my things, and headed toward the office. Every time I came here, I was glad my physiotherapist was located in a business area. When you live in a German city, you always have to street park because there's never a designated parking lot. Except if you went to a business area. When I went inside, New York had already slipped my mind.

When I got back to my car, it was 3:47 p.m. Not the time for the news yet, but they were still talking about New York on the radio. A second plane had crashed into the other Twin Tower of the World

Trade Center. More smoke, explosions, confusion, and the first speculations that this wasn't an accident but an act of terror. When I got home, I turned on the TV.

This Tuesday, that had started with sunshine and such good news, turned out to be one of the darkest days in human history. I don't need to describe any details; we all still see the horrible pictures of that day, just hearing the date, 9/11. But I also learned something that day: humility.

From the day that I had walked out of my educational psychology lesson and had sat on that bench beside the university's beat-up basketball court, I had felt like I owned a monopoly on misery. Nobody had a tougher life than I had. Nobody was facing a bigger surgery than I did. And nobody could compete with the injustice of the number of bad things that had happened to me. Fucking no one.

Sitting in my living room that day, watching the Twin Towers collapse over and over again in a rerun, my misery suddenly felt benign. My believed injustice felt like a toddler tantrum compared to what was going on, on the other side of the world. Who was I thinking I had it bad in life? I had people around me who loved me, who were ready to do close to anything to save my life. If I'd die, I'd die because of a disease, surrounded by love, not because of hate.

When Aria and I finally turned off the TV and went to bed that night, I knew I should consider myself lucky. There were so many good things in my life, and at least for this one day, I was able to appreciate them.

The days ticked by. October was almost done, the first Christmas cookies had made an appearance on the shelves of every supermarket, but still no organs in sight. I had already waited for almost two months, and with every day that passed by, I realized I couldn't wait any longer. It drove me nuts that I didn't know how long I had to wait. If I had known I had to wait four more weeks, I would have waited patiently. But waking up every morning, knowing this could be the day, and then going to bed that night, knowing this hadn't been the day, was dreadful.

In addition to all of that, my health was also not in the mood for waiting any longer. It declined day by day. Every day I felt like a tiny piece of my body, my so-called temple, fell off and shattered into a million pieces at my feet. Never replaced.

One morning, Aria even asked me about it.

"Did you cough all night?" she asked while starting the coffee machine with a big yawn. "I thought I heard you a few times. Sounded horrible."

"Yeah, I did cough a lot. I'm sorry." I sat down at our kitchen table, watching her. Her vibrant curly hair, the healthy curves of her body, her energy, her health. *Verdammt.*

"Are you still walking the dog today?" The coffee machine began to brew as she sat down.

"Yes," I said. "Like, every morning. Keeps my lungs breathing."

I didn't want to tell her that I had started skipping a few morning walks here and there. It was just too exhausting. Walking suddenly felt like sprinting. I huffed like I was ascending the Alps. Every time I got home after a walk, I felt like I wanted to sleep till the next morning. Or even better, sleep until the day of my transplant. Escape the depression of witnessing my slow decay and not being able to do anything about it.

"Maybe you shouldn't walk and stay home. Rest a little. Catch up on sleep. Coffee?" The pot was almost filled to the top. Bless God for caffeine.

"Yes, thank you," I said.

She placed the mug in front of me and sat down again. She still had some time before she had to go to university and live her healthy life.

"I know," I yawned in between two sips. "I should move my body. It's good for me, but on the other hand, yeah, I am tired. Tired of it all actually. Tired of waiting, of fighting all the time. Tired of living a life that doesn't even feel like mine anymore. Man, I wish I could go to university. Being bored there instead of here."

"Remember we have tickets for the Chinese National Circus next week? That's something to look forward to. I know I am. For sure better than the marketing lecture I'll have to sit through this morning."

"True," I said, but the tickets weren't able to cheer me up. I had wanted to go see the circus, and I still did, but one show of the Chinese National Circus was not enough to give me the feeling of being alive. I wanted to do so much more. Circus, movies, meeting friends, going out, running with the dog—my list was endless. But all I could do was wait and go see one show. Witnessing one tightrope dance while hoping not to fall off myself.

Soon after Aria left for university, I took care of some emails my friends had sent as a response to the email I had sent weeks ago, telling them how I had still believed I needed a liver transplant.

I had also gotten some phone calls, but whatever medium my friends chose, all of them read and sounded the same: somewhat helpless.

Nobody knew what to tell me. How to cheer me up, or how to convey hope. What do you say to someone who's facing probable death at the age of twenty-two?

"It will be fine."

"You of all people will make it."

"You will be healthy again in no time."

"Dying is not an option."

Geez, even I didn't know.

Besides hollow get-well-card phrases and my reassuring everyone it would all be fine, there wasn't much exchange between me and my friends. Not via phone, nor via emails. Nobody knew what to say. Nobody knew how to deal with me, least of all myself. Did I want to hear what my friends were doing? If they had fallen in love or recently out of? I didn't know. I didn't ask, and none of my friends dared to share their normality with me. The Inka I had been a few months ago wasn't there anymore. Once I might have been compassionate, caring, and fun to be around, but not anymore. I just didn't have the strength to goof around, to laugh, to call back and ask how everything was going. All the strength I still had was reserved for myself. I had one goal: to survive my own death, and I was ready to give it my all. I had become a blunt, selfish, and exhausted person. Everything I did, I did for myself. The emails I wrote back to my friends were only filled with my stuff. I asked no questions about how they were doing; I didn't care. I didn't have the energy to care. It was rough seeing myself vanish and not feeling like Inka anymore. I truly hoped Inka would come back once I got transplanted. If I'd ever get transplanted.

I sent another email, this one to a friend I had known since elementary school. This email was filled with nothing but selfishness too. Me, me, and some more of me, but not even one of my friends complained about it. A true friend stays by your side even when you're at your worst. I was, and they all did.

My mom called shortly after. Just to hear how I was doing, how my night had been, the usual motherly stuff.

"I'm good," I lied. "Night was okay. I'll soon take a walk with Fenja, eat lunch— oh, and next week we're going to the Chinese National Circus. Can't wait."

More lies.

"Oh, the Circus, right," my mom said, and then after a short moment of silence: "You sound breathless. Have you been moving around or are your lungs getting worse? You know, we can always call the doctors in Hannover. Maybe get you some antibiotics?"

"I've been moving around. Emptying the . . . the dishwasher," I lied again.

I didn't want to lie to my mom, or to my parents in general, but admitting to them that I was out of breath from just sitting around writing emails wasn't going to happen either. I didn't want them to worry more than they did, and I didn't want to admit to myself how fast my health was running out on me. I'd get a new set of lungs, eventually. Who cared about the original one? It was all good. All. Good.

"Hmm," was her response. Not believing a single word I said, but also not calling me out on it. Instead, she asked: "Are you using the oxygen during the day now?"

"I do," I said, "mostly in the evening while watching TV." And this time I was telling the truth. I was using oxygen more and more. In the beginning, I had only used it during the night, but now I put it on as often as possible. Another sad example for my current situation.

"That's good," my mom said. I could almost see her nodding along, affirming to herself how everything was grand with her youngest daughter. I wasn't the only one who could lie to herself.

"Ahem . . ." I cleared my throat. "I actually wanna get going, with the dog, outside. That's why I—"

My mom immediately got the hint.

"Oh yeah, I'm sorry. You go outside. I just wanted to check in. Your dad says hi too. He's preparing a package for you with books he thought you might like. To keep the boredom away . . . Anyway, we will talk tomorrow. We love you, and put on a jacket when you go outside. One thing you don't need right now is a cold."

"Love you guys too," I answered with a verbally added rolling of my eyes. My parents and the jacket. According to them, every virus could be fought off by just wearing a jacket. No matter the weather, a jacket was my ultimate protection against the flu, a cold, pneumonia—you name it.

"Kisses to Dad, and we talk tomorrow. Byeee."

We hung up, and I immediately felt bad for not telling her the truth. Why did I have to lie about my nights that were filled with coughing galore and how breathing had become a constant struggle? I was listed for a lung and liver transplant for God's sake. I had the right to feel bad, I was required to feel bad to be on the waiting list, and I still tried to make myself look healthy in front of my parents. As if I could trick them into believing their daughter was anything but dying. Ridiculous.

I went to take the dog out but only to pee, not for a walk. When I was back inside, again sitting at my desk as if I were the busiest pencil pusher on the planet, I decided to write another letter, an actual letter filled with nothing but the truth. And there was only one person I could send such an honest letter to:

> Dear Ingo,
>
> Another letter from me because today everything is just fucked and I need a shoulder to cry on. During the night, I couldn't sleep because I coughed all the time.

Thanks to my pee pill, my stomach is now flat, but the mucus in my lungs is even thicker. If you extract liquid from the body, it also kind of dries out the mucus. My lungs are painful from all the coughing, as well as my head. I'm tired and in a bad mood as usual. And in addition, my damn blood sugar is acting crazy. If I want normal blood sugar levels, I need to eat less. But I can't eat less because I need to gain weight. Damn, everything is just bleh. Beside feeling like shit, I'm also waiting like a crazy person for my phone to ring to finally get notified: They have organs for me. I'm sure it will ring this month. If not, I must stop thinking about it. Otherwise, I will also get to know the psychiatric wing of the Hannover Medical School.

I want it to ring, and on the other hand, I'm afraid it might ring when I'm not feeling well. I can't survive a double lung and liver transplant when I already feel like shit. And then I'm afraid it'll ring when I'm feeling great because then it'll feel like I'm not ready to be transplanted yet.

And you know what? I don't have the energy anymore to fight myself back up again. My health went up and down so many times during the last few months. I don't wanna keep dragging my damaged lungs out of the mud anymore. I want to exchange them and fight with a new perspective.

Yes, for sure you are right when you say I try to will my

phone to ring. You don't have to tell me it isn't a good idea. That I must stop doing it. I know.

Is it easier to deal with the certainty of death than with the uncertainty of it? I mean, I'm glad I have at least a second chance. You didn't have that. Death was certain for you. But then I also think it might be easier to prepare yourself for death only than preparing yourself for both life and death. It kills me not to know what will be. — Your I-am-so-done-with-it-all-and-drowning-in-self-pity niece

7

Meet Martina

December 7—which marked my three months of waiting time—came and went. No phone call. No organs. Nothing.

I was so angry. All the time. Had God or whoever was responsible for organ distribution up there just forgotten about me? Why did I have to wait so long? Why couldn't I just get transplanted and move on? Why did I have to suffer for so long? Hadn't I already suffered enough? If anyone deserved new organs, it was me. Fucking me and no one else.

Not to lose my mind, and not to lose my friends due to my exceptionally inviting mood, I tried to keep myself busy during the weeks before Christmas. I crafted, I made three saint kings out of clay, colored them in detail, baked, wrote a Christmas story, and collected premonitions. Fiercely.

My sister dreamed I'd get transplanted in the week of December 10. I marked it in my calendar.

My roommate had a feeling it might happen the Monday after—calendar.

My grandmother's move to a senior citizen home was complete, so now was the right time—calendar.

I had finally read the last pages of the never-ending book *The Pope's Rhinoceros*, so I was ready. Thus, calendar. But nothing moved.

Everything stood still, frozen in time. As if I were still sitting in the examination room of the liver transplant department, hearing about my upcoming transplant, but nobody had hit the play button. Maybe nobody had even realized that I was still sitting there, glued to that awful plastic chair, trying to move on but being unable to. After all, everyone else seemed to continue living. Everyone around me planned their Christmas holidays, bought presents, looked forward to Hallmark movies, hot chocolate, and a joyous time. Everyone but me. I just couldn't. I didn't want to buy presents, I didn't want to get any either, and I didn't want to celebrate and pretend to be happy and jolly, when all I wanted, all I deserved in life, was denied.

Eventually, I decided to stay glued to that examination room chair of the liver transplant department, keep the pause button pressed, and not celebrate Christmas this year. I didn't want to celebrate anything. I was too stubborn. If I didn't get new organs, screw it, I wouldn't celebrate Christmas either. I wouldn't participate in life at all before I got a new one. That's why I didn't spend the holidays with my family, but with a good friend of mine, Martina.

In the mid-1960s, when my mom was still an active swimmer, she trained every day at the pool. Her lifeguard, Horst Ritscher, always made sure my mom had her own lane. He also ensured no one would disturb her training or splash or breathe the wrong way around her. He was proud to take care of her because my mom was not only swimming lap after lap, but she was also training to qualify for the next Olympic games. In 1968, she would be part of the German Olympic swim team, winning a bronze medal in Mexico City.

All summer she spent at the pool, talking to Horst every day. When his daughter Martina was born, Mom graciously accepted the title of godmother.

Years later, Martina became an unofficial godmother to me. A friend but also my rock in times of need. Just like Christmas 2001.

Martina lived about half an hour from where I lived, in Bremen. Bremen is not very known overseas. It's a small, picturesque city, its population only about 500,000, about the same as it was in 2001, but still, most people have at least heard of it through the tale from the Grimm brothers called *Town Musicians of Bremen*. The main characters of said tale even have a bronze statue standing at Bremen's market square—a donkey, with a dog, cat, and rooster stacked on top of it. The donkey's hooves and nose are polished to gold from being touched for luck since 1953. The protector of the city is called Roland, and he can also be found in the market square.

At first sight, Roland doesn't look all that impressive besides his height of eighteen feet. A gray statue, looking nothing like a protector with his boyish face and cute locks, holding a sword and a shield, crowned by a baldachin. But he's been here since 1404, keeps an eye on the city hall that was added in 2004, same as Roland, to the list of UNESCO World Heritage Sites. Some believe the city hall is the most beautiful building in Bremen. With its ornate gothic architecture, I can agree. My heart had always belonged to Oldenburg, but Bremen was like a city out of a German fairytale.

When I arrived in Bremen on the afternoon of Christmas Eve at Martina's terraced house, she opened the door and gave me a long, heartfelt hug.

"Hello, my Inka-Kind," she said, her nickname for me, Inka-child.

"Merry Christmas," I said in return and handed her the bag of stuff I had brought with me. I was exhausted. Half an hour driving, carrying the bag from my door to my car, and now from my car to her door was almost too much for me.

Martina wore her hair even shorter than my mom, as if she was ready to join the military by the end of the holidays. She looked tough. As straightforward as she was, only her big-rimmed, fire-red glasses softened her appearance a bit, same as her warm smile. She took my jacket and the bag, then pointed toward the kitchen.

"Can you smell it?" she asked. "Do you know what I'm making?"

"Ehhh, no?" I took my shoes off, common practice in Germany when entering someone's home, and walked into the kitchen. The smell, and moreover the sight, was intoxicatingly delicious.

Martina rushed ahead of me and pointed at the dim spotlight inside the boiling hot oven.

"Christmas goose," she exclaimed. "It's almost done."

She opened the oven for a split second, and the kitchen filled with a hot cloud of butter-roasted thyme, rosemary, and apples. My stomach growled.

"With it we will have potato dumplings aaaand . . ." She lifted the lid from one of the pots on the stove. "Gravy. Gallons of gravy. What do you say?"

"I'm hungry," I said with a huge smile on my face. "And I'm impressed. I never had Christmas goose. Not even for Christmas."

"Well, you never spend Christmas with me. That's why." She grinned. "Let's set the table. Food is almost ready. I'm hungry too—oh, and merry Christmas."

It was great spending the holidays with Martina. It felt special, because of the food, the peace and quiet, our late-night TV marathons while lying in bed, and eating even more food, but it didn't feel so Christmassy that I felt sad for not being home with my family.

On my last day at Martina's, I sat upstairs in her upper living room, dogs and pillows surrounding me. With her two pugs at my side, I finally decided to follow a suggestion she had made over Christmas goose and potato dumpling to help me cope with the endless waiting time: to write a wish list for my life after transplant.

"First of all, you love to write," she had said. "And you are so good at it. So far, I loved everything you've written. Everything! But now it's time to write something solely for yourself. A wish list for the life after will give you something specific to wait for, not just empty time. You will get an idea what you are fighting for, why it's worth it to keep going. More gravy?"

I nodded and leaned back so she could drown my dumplings once again in sauce.

"So, what do you say?" she asked.

"Thank you for the compliment, and it's delicious!" I said with a full mouth.

"I'm talking about the wish list for your new life, dummy. If you want something, you need to know what you want it for. You can't just hope for a new life while not having any idea what you want it for."

"More time?" I said tentatively. I had no idea what exactly I wanted to do if I'd ever get transplanted. I didn't dare look to the future—maybe there was none—but Martina didn't have any of it.

"Inka-Kind, seriously, you gotta look ahead. Your approach is nothing but wishy-washy, nor here, nor there. You need to know what you are fighting for, or this"—she pointed at me—"won't work. Get out of here, you little bugger!" she suddenly shouted, shooing one of her pugs out of the dining room. "Think about it." She looked at me again. "I know I'm right. Writing is going to save you. Another dumpling?"

This was Martina, gruff and warmhearted, two for the price of one. But even now, a few days later, I still wasn't sure of it at all, but ready to give it a try. A wish list for my life after transplant. After all, I always loved to write.

At first, it was not easy for me to think ahead. Not only because I had no idea of how my life after transplant would look like, but also because I had never really thought ahead. Even before I knew I needed a transplant, I had never come up with any wishes of how my future should look like. Never. Even today, I'm not planning ahead much. My future always looked and looks like a blank piece of paper. It is there, I'm planning on living it, but it has to draw itself naturally and on its own.

But here I was, sitting in the corner of Martina's sofa, the snorting of her two pugs in my ears, trying to come up with milestones for my healthy life 2.0.

And it felt weird.

I chewed through two pencils and about twenty cookies before I was ready to write down the first non-monumental item for my wish list: I wanted to celebrate the Christmas I had just refused to celebrate some day in the future. I also wanted to have a party, a post-transplant party, with all my friends. Then go on vacation, get a second dog, buy new clothes, start running again, maybe even a marathon, finish my psychology degree . . .

All the items on my wish list turned out to be non-monumental. Did I want to do something exceptional in the future? Sure. But at that moment, exceptional meant nothing but being healthy. All I wanted, all I could come up with, was a normal, healthy life. Waking up every morning and being able to breathe. Go on a vacation, exercise a little, be a psychologist, and play with my two dogs. I couldn't come up with anything better than that.

I didn't share my wish list with anyone out of fear that no one would be able to value my dreams as much as I did. Wishing for being able to breathe in the morning, during exercise, and in the evening seemed lame. Only that . . . it wasn't. By wishing to be healthy, I actually wished for the impossible.

The goal after transplant was to be functional again. To be able to live for five more years. To be able to enjoy a little bit more time. But I didn't want that. I wanted to be healthy. I wanted to be breathing, I wanted to be free of physical limitations, and free to do anything I could dream of. Because without breath, it was baffling how little was possible. Without breath, everything became a thing. Even things like walking up the stairs. Climbing stairs was nothing I did without thinking about it. It was a task that had to be tackled with determination, coughing, and exhaustion. Grocery shopping—the same. Walking the dog—the same. Doing laundry—same. Just imagining doing laundry without even thinking about it, throwing the clothes into the washing machine, then throwing them into the dryer, and then doing other things because laundry wouldn't exhaust me was intoxicating.

That's exactly what I wanted: health. And all the possibilities that came with it.

When I got back home the next day, I sat down at my desk and wrote another letter to Ingo. I had to share my excitement. I had to allow myself to bubble over . . . but only to him:

Dear Ingo,

Guess what I did yesterday? Well, I'm sure you know

already. From where you're sitting, you can probably see everything, but I still want to tell you: I wrote a wish list! A wish list for my new life. Even though it wasn't easy to let go of the question of when my phone would finally ring and think about my future instead. It took me some time to let go, but I have to say, now, since it's done and the wish list lays in front of me, it felt good writing it. It reminds me why I'm doing all this bullshit in the first place. That there might be more than light at the end of the tunnel.

Next, I want to write my will, and I have to say, it seems weird to me to write a will at all. I know, I said I want to prepare myself for life *and* death, but it's still a completely different feeling writing a wish list for your new life or a will for your upcoming death. It's scary. Like bad karma. Did you have a similar feeling when you wrote your will? Weren't you afraid to only invite death by writing about it?

On the other hand, I have to say, because of your will, it feels as if you tricked death in the end. You are still, at least sometimes, alive, and part of our lives. My mom still uses your leather wiener-dog key chain. She probably doesn't think of you every time she holds it, but for sure sometimes. And I can't even count how often my dad told the story of how he tried, after your death, to fix the adventurous electric cable constructions in the bus you left for him. And myself, and the letter you wrote to me . . . I don't think I'd be sitting here,

> writing these words to you, if it wasn't for that letter. You see, twenty-two years later, and we still think of you.
>
> Okay, I'll write a will. I can't resist. I also want to pull one over on death at least once. — Your from-all-the-wishing-she's-almost-drunk niece

The year 2001 ended in the company of friends and a glass of nonalcoholic sparkling wine in my hand. It probably was the best alternative to what I had wished for: to spend New Year's Eve in the hospital, in ICU, recovering from my transplant.

8

Crappy New Year

The New Year started, and sickness welcomed me with open arms, a running nose, congested lungs, and a banner over my head that read: Crappy New Year! It would have been a normal cold for everyone else, but for me it was a full-grown respiratory infection that had to be treated with intravenous antibiotics. The only good thing about it: I could do it all from home.

For fourteen days, I'd get two antibiotic infusions every eight hours that would help eliminate all the bacteria rummaging through my lungs. The infusions were delivered to my home and took up most of our fridge space and most of the fridge space of our neighbors. I'd connect and disconnect them as needed. I knew how to take care of an infusion like other girls knew how to apply nail polish. I knew how to keep everything sterile and how to flush my IV; I'd been my own nurse for long enough. The only thing I couldn't do by myself was place a new venous access when the old one was done. For that I had to go to the hospital.

A venous access is a thin plastic catheter, like a syringe, that's inserted into the vein and stays there for multiple days. Through this tiny plastic catheter, the infusions would be administered.

Unfortunately, no venous access lasts fourteen days of IV therapy. Normally, after three to four days of usage, the vein the catheter was inserted in would get infected from the aggressive antibiotics and a new venous access would be placed. And that almost always happened over the weekend, and always around nighttime.

This time, it was a Saturday, 10:30 p.m. when my venous access decided it had had enough and wouldn't let anything go through it anymore.

For a short moment I considered to just screw it, pull the old catheter out, apply a Band-Aid, go to bed, skip the last two infusions of the day, and drive to the hospital first thing in the morning to get a new venous access placed. But I didn't. Skipping a dosage of antibiotics was never a good idea. The bacteria in my lungs could build up an antimicrobial resistance, learning how to defeat the drugs that were destined to kill them, and make my life even harder.

I sighed. I knew what I had to do.

I went to talk to Aria.

"What's up?" she asked when I came to her room. Aria looked at my exposed catheter, the tube attached to it just dangling down my arm, without any infusion connected to it. "Don't tell me we have to go to the hospital now to get you a new access?"

Obviously, this wasn't the first time the two of us drove to the hospital to get me hooked up again. But it was the first time in the middle of the night. I knew what we were up against, showing up at the hospital at this hour: my regular doctor at home, enjoying his emergency-free evening, and the doctor on call not knowing what to do. Aria on the other hand had never been in an ER at this hour, as her ER experience was solely based on the TV series with the same name, which I was willing to use for my advantage.

"Will you join me?" I asked.

"Sure." She smiled, turned off the TV, and got off the couch. "Give me just one second. I have to change out of my PJs first. You never know, there might be cute doctors."

As I said, she had no idea. I knew there weren't any but didn't want to dampen her enthusiasm for going to the hospital at night. While she changed, I went to the bathroom, pulled the old catheter out of my arm, and applied a Band-Aid. I didn't change. Instead, I covered up my PJs with a long coat. Good enough. Especially for the doctors I knew we would see tonight.

We drove to the old children's hospital in Oldenburg. Old, because it was established in 1953. A new extension to the old building was supposed to open in 2003, but for now this was the only place to go; plus, I liked going there because the old children's hospital didn't have an ER. I wouldn't have to compete with people who had broken limbs or were about to die from a heart attack. It would only be me and hopefully a cooperative doctor.

We parked at the entrance of the hospital, in one of the ten parking spots that were available for visitors, and went to see the gatekeeper, a security guard who watched the hospital's entrance at night and decided who was allowed inside and who wasn't. As I said, it was the *old* children's hospital.

The gatekeeper was sitting in a tiny, dark booth right beside the main door, looking up from a car magazine when he saw us coming.

"Yes?" he asked through the little window of his booth.

"Good evening. I'm here to get a new venous access placed in my arm. I'm doing intravenous therapy at home, antibiotics via infusions," I clarified, "but my catheter broke, and I need it replaced by the doctor who's on call tonight. I'm also a patient here. There should be a chart somewhere confirming what I'm saying."

The confused gatekeeper buzzed the door open and told us to wait inside the building for a nurse to come see us.

Step one: accomplished. We were inside the hospital. Next step would be to convince the nurse to let us see the doctor. I crossed my fingers she wouldn't be anything like Nurse Ratched.

The entrance hall looked more like a train station than a hospital. High ceilings, a huge staircase winding up toward the first floor, and dark, stone floor under our feet.

"Creepy," Aria said, and she was right. It looked like the halls of an abandoned mental hospital. Only the smell of popcorn and the cackling of a clown were missing.

We didn't have to wait long until the nurse came down the staircase. She was wearing a colorful top with blue pants, like a modern children's hospital nurse, but if she had been in a white uniform and a white hat, just like Nurse Ratched, I wouldn't have been surprised.

"How can I help you?" she asked with a pinched face and sharp tone the moment she came to a stop in front of us.

I explained quickly why I needed a new venous access placed in my arm, and that I needed it right now—not tomorrow, not in the morning, now.

"We can't just place a venous access into a person's arm and let them go home with it," she told me matter-of-factly. "Who's the doctor you see here at the hospital?" She had started to tap her foot with impatience, but I decided to ignore it. I'd get my new venous access, one way or the other.

"I see Dr. K here at the hospital. He's the only CF doctor here," I answered matter-of-factly, mimicking her drill sergeant tone. "He's the doctor who oversees my intensive, fourteen-day, intravenous antibiotic therapy. Which I do *at home,*" I added with maybe a little too much force. "And to be able to administer the last dose of antibiotics for today at home, I need a new catheter."

I reached into my bag and pulled out one of the infusions to show her I wasn't making this up.

Her eyebrows raised. I was sure she had never seen an at-home infusion. They looked different than the ones at the hospital. My infusions weren't plastic bags that had to be hung on an infusion stand; mine were shaped like little hand grenades. Inside the transparent grenade was a balloon filled with medication, the grenade itself was under pressure, and when released, it would press the medication into the patient's vein. No need to hang them anywhere. You could put them in your pocket while the medication ran through if you wanted to.

Her eyes shifted away from the grenade and back to me.

"Can I see the venous access that isn't working anymore?"

I should have known this was coming. At home, I had even thought for a second about leaving the old one inside my arm as proof, but when it came to hospital rules, I couldn't resist defying them.

I pulled up my sleeve and exposed the Band-Aid.

"I pulled it at home," I said.

"Only medical personnel are allowed to pull a venous access," she scolded me, also not the first time I heard that one. I wanted to tell her how pulling a catheter from your own arm wasn't rocket science, a monkey could have done it, but I didn't. Like so often, best things go unsaid.

I just shrugged and pulled my sleeve back down.

She shrugged too, then shook her head as if to let me know how tiring it was to deal with patients like me, patients who thought they knew everything better, and then waved us to follow her.

"It might take some time before the doctor is ready to see you," she told us over her shoulder, then rushed up the stairs, leaving us in her wake.

We sat on hard plastic chairs in a hall, closed doors to our right and left, waiting for the doctor to show up. I was glad to be sitting. Rushing up the stairs had taken every breath from me. I already felt better because of the antibiotics I had been taking the last few days, but I was still waiting for a lung transplant, and it showed.

"You okay?" Aria asked.

"Yeah, just give me a second."

It was only us sitting in the hall, the humming fluorescent lights above, and my huffing filling the silence.

"I don't know," Aria said after a while. "In the show *ER*, there's always action. Always a cute doctor rushing by, a hot nurse. This . . . "—she spread her arms—"is hugely disappointing."

I wanted to say, "I could have warned you," but as if he heard us, one of the doors to our left opened and a doctor stepped out. Aria immediately sat upright, but it was more reflex than necessity. He was young, that much I was able to give him, but other than that reminded me a lot more of *ER*'s Dr. Greene than of Dr. Ross. Thinning hairline, askew glasses, and dark rings under his eyes.

He yawned, then came toward us, took off his glasses, and cleaned them with the corner of his white coat. "Hi, I'm Dr. B. How can I help you?"

I had assumed he already knew from the nurse who had brought us up here why I was sitting in his hall, waiting to see him, but no. I had to explain a third time why I was there. When I was done, Dr. B looked at me, put his glasses back on, then looked at Aria, then me again, and shook his head.

"We can't just place a venous access into a patient's arm and let them go home with it," he said.

Fucking déjà vu.

"I know," I said. "The nurse had said something similar, but I do need a new access, otherwise I won't be able to administer the two antibiotic infusions I still need for tonight."

Since we had this conversation already once, Aria saw it as her cue to pull out my infusions and show them to our doctor.

He reached for one of the hand grenades, read the label, noted the doctor's name on it who prescribed it to me, and gave it back to me.

"And Dr. K. is a physician in this hospital?" he asked.

I nodded. I didn't roll my eyes, which took immense stamina. "He's at the pulmonary department. Taking care of the CF patients."

"Can I see the venous access you have right now? The one that isn't working?"

I looked over to Aria. She looked at me, and I knew we both had the same thought: This was what *Candid Camera* must have felt like. Ordinary people being confronted with unusually stupid situations.

"I pulled it at home," I said with a shrug. I didn't pull up my sleeve this time.

"Only medical personnel are allowed to pull a venous access."

"I know." I wanted to scream down the empty hall: "Just fucking put a new catheter in my arm!" But again, I didn't.

Eventually, the young doctor with the askew glasses brought back the nurse from earlier and asked her to place a new venous access into my arm. She might not have been the friendliest, but she knew how to put a needle in someone's arm. Ten minutes later, we were back in the car. My first infusion was already running through my vein while Aria drove us home. We joked a little bit about how I had to explain everything three times. How we both could have stayed in our PJs and how a hospital clown, walking the halls at night, trying to rip people's arms off, would have made our visit so much more memorable, but okay, at least we were back home not too late in the morning hours. Not bad at all, considering the task at hand, but I still felt beyond exhausted. It was not only the IV therapy itself. Having hardcore antibiotics pumped into my system, three times a day, was exhausting on its own. It was also the situation itself that had drained me.

I had no problem telling doctors what they had to do, to argue with them, and stand my ground. I had done it from an early age on. Had always been an advocate for myself, but no matter how tough I looked on the outside, on the inside, there was always worry. What if the doctor wouldn't place a new catheter in my arm? What if he refused to let me go home with a catheter? What if he decided to go by the rules, send me to a real ER at a different hospital, and let them decide if I truly needed IVs or not? Would I even be able to do something like that, considering my declined health and broken body?

It's not that I would have been in danger if I had missed my night antibiotics. After all, I even had considered skipping them myself. No big deal, but on the other hand . . . it was. This was *my* health, this was *my* life I tried to hold on to—and still, I depended on doctors helping me on my journey. Staying healthy was not only my decision, but it also depended on the doctors' decisions. That scared me. There were so many *what ifs*, and if a doctor decided to go against my wishes, there was absolutely nothing I could do about it.

When I was a young teenager, I was in the hospital once due to a lung infection. I was on a very high dose of oral antibiotics—very high for normal patients, not for CF patients—and the doctor at the hospital refused to give me such a high dose under his watch. He simply didn't know much about cystic fibrosis, as it wasn't common around 1995.

I called my mom that evening, as she had already gone home, and told her through tears how they wouldn't give me the medication I needed. I was terrified my lungs would take a toll if not treated properly. Here I was, knowing what had to be done, but being refused of it. I couldn't force the doctor to give me the right meds, I couldn't prescribe them myself, I couldn't do anything but sit there and watch my lungs decline. I considered pressing my call button again to ask to see the doctor one more time; once he'd enter, I would throw the antibiotics at him, and they'd bounce off his unknowledgeable forehead. But my education prevented me from doing any such thing. My throwing skills as well. *Arschloch.* Asshole.

I was released the next day. When I was back home, I continued taking the right dosage of antibiotics. Two missed doses didn't have any effect on my lungs. It was all good—only the fear of something like that ever happening again stuck around. And I had felt it tonight.

Two days later, I was again back at the same hospital, only this time it was a scheduled visit. I was *invited* to stay five nights with the endocrinologists to have my blood sugar adjusted. It was still close to impossible for me to find the right amount of insulin I needed to contain a normal blood sugar level. I was always either too low or too high. I either had to gobble up anything sweet, *fast*, so as not to collapse from too low blood sugar, or I had to skip food because I first had to wait for my blood sugar to go down again.

It was a constant struggle I had to get under control because it prevented me from gaining weight, and weight I had to gain with

5″6′ and 88 pounds. I was running the risk of being taken off the transplant list because I was almost too skinny to be able to survive a transplant. Hopefully the endocrinologists could help. They were assigned to teach me more about diabetes itself, and what nutrition I should eat to keep my blood sugar low and my calorie intake high.

My sister came over to help take care of my dog and to bring me my IV infusions every day to the hospital. The endocrinology department's fridge wasn't big enough to store everyone's insulin and my IVs.

At least this time it was easy to convince the nurses and doctors to allow me to take care of my antibiotic therapy myself. I wasn't ready to give any of my responsibility to nurses who were specialized in diabetic care, and the nurses weren't ready to take any of my responsibility in return. It was perfect. I was able to concentrate solely on my diabetes, no arguing with nurses or doctors—well, almost no arguing, until the third day of my diabetes training.

My morning nurse and I had already established a routine. Around 6:00 a.m., she'd bring me my antibiotic infusions that my sister had dropped off the day before. I'd get my IV running and enjoy another half hour in bed until my nurse would come in again at around 6:30 to officially start the day for me. Only this morning was different. When my nurse came into my room again, breakfast in tow, I told her: "I can't eat breakfast this morning. I have an EGD scheduled at eight, down with the gastroenterologists."

An EGD, or esophagogastroduodenoscopy, is an endoscopy of the esophagus and the stomach. To have this done, I'd get a tube guided through my mouth, down my esophagus, all the way to my stomach while being sedated.

The reason why I needed this procedure was esophageal varices. The varices were a side effect of my liver cirrhosis and could potentially be fatal if they decided to burst.

When I was ten, I had a severe case of burst varices and internal bleeding. I got multiple blood transfusions and thankfully made it through. To prevent it from happening again, I had to undergo an EGD every year to seal the varices that looked like they might burst. So far it had worked, and I was not ready to postpone my upcoming EGD solely because of diabetes training.

My nurse first couldn't believe she hadn't been informed up front of my appointment with gastro, but then agreed with me how miscommunication between the different departments had probably been the culprit, even though it wasn't. I had just kept it all to myself.

Of course, the EGD could have been re-scheduled for another time, and it probably should have. There was no reason to cram everything I had going on in one week's time. IV antibiotics, diabetes training, *and* EGD. Though the honest answer was a bit different. First, I wanted to be done with everything as quickly as possible and therefore had decided not to reschedule and also hadn't told anyone about it so no one could make me reschedule. Second, my stubbornness. I didn't reschedule because I wanted to show to myself and anyone else how I was still totally capable of handling IV therapy, diabetes training, and EGD at the same time. Capable in a sense of still being fit enough to get through it. If I could do this, I couldn't be as sick as I felt. If I could do it, I could do everything else as well. Including a triple organ transplant. As long as my head believed in my health, my body would follow suit.

I got back to my room around 11:00 a.m. The EGD had been eventless, two varices had been sealed, and soon they'd bring lunch. My next diabetes lesson was at 2:00 p.m. Till then, my head would hopefully be clear again after the sedation and I'd be ready to go. The only bad thing: I had missed the visit of my sister, but she had left me a letter. A typical *my sister* letter:

> Good morning, dearest sister of mine!
>
> Keep going and don't anger the nurses so much. I heard all about you ditching diabetes training this morning just to have some fun with the gastroenterologists instead. She did not like it. But I made sure you'll get lunch later. I know, I'm the best sister ever.
>
> Anyway, you can't relax for much longer in your sterile hospital bed, we can't afford that—you must pay co-pay now. Put some pressure on your varices and don't let anyone peek inside of you.
>
> I hope I'll see you tonight and not only tomorrow morning because I have (drum roll) a PRESENT for you. I was thinking maybe a huge box of chocolate or a fat ice cream. To see how well you can measure the right amount of insulin after all the training you got. Yes, I've always been very sensitive and creative in these kinds of situations. Your infusions for today are in the nurse's fridge BTW. All set and ready.
>
> Big hug from me, and wet licks from Fenja and Aimee!
>
> Your favorite sister! [I only have one]

My IV-therapy-diabetes-training-EGD marathon was done, and my sister was glad to be on her way back home. It had been exhausting, for both of us. I might have tricked myself into believing I was still healthy, resilient, and strong, because I had survived this one week of crazy, but during the quiet hours of my evenings, I could admit to myself that I wasn't as resilient anymore as I liked to seem. The IV therapy had helped me to feel better, sure, but my overall energy level struggled to recover. The walks with my dog were short. More and more often I plugged the oxygen under my nose, sometimes even during the day, and whenever Aria invited me to do something with her, I struggled to find enthusiasm for it.

While my evenings were truth ridden, my days were not. During the day, I was always able to convince myself that I wasn't low on energy at all. I was great. I could breathe better, I coughed less, and there was no CF patient in the world who had survived a week like I had, who still walked their dog every day, while being listed for a lung and liver transplant. Not only were my days clouded by my unshakable belief that I was still doing great, but my dreams were clouded too.

January 22, 2002

Last night I had a really cool dream. I was in the hospital because of my transplant. It was after the operation. I woke up and was completely surprised. It all went perfectly. The operation had only taken four hours, I had no pain, and was already able to stand up carefully. First, my legs were a little numb, like they had fallen asleep, but that went away pretty quickly. I walked up and down the halls and was able to breathe normally. I was only afraid to touch my stomach because of the Band-Aid on and the scar under it. But the operation was a full success. I had even forgotten to let everyone know because it had been such a benign event.

During this time of me flying high and seeing the world through rose-colored glasses, I finally found the courage to write my last will.

9

LAST WILL & TESTAMENT

Inviting death over to spend a few hours with me was actually less painful than having to deal with doctors—of any kind. Preparing myself for death might have seemed scary at first, but very quickly it turned . . . well, fun.

I took an empty composition book I still had lying around inside a desk drawer, decorated the cover with a postcard showing a hearse pulling empty cans after it, similar to a wedding car, and a sign attached to the bumper saying: Just died!

I knew my mom would not be amused if she ever had to see my last will decorated by black humor, but I also knew my sister would. Death required some humor. There was no way around it.

As a former student, not having any kind of job, solely living from the support my parents were able to provide, I had no money to leave behind. My will was all about the small, everyday items I owned. Mementos I had collected throughout my life and now hoped would help my friends to remember me when I was gone.

First, I walked around my apartment, opened boxes, drawers, shoe cartons, anything I hadn't looked into for years to make some kind of inventory. Once that was done, I sat down, opened the composition book destined to carry my will, and assigned my mementos to the people I loved most in this world. And with every name I jotted down,

I truly felt more and more prepared for death. I couldn't imagine a better way to plan my departure. Ingo had been a good example.

I could see Lydia's face, when she would receive my white stuffed seal animal called Fridolin. Lydia was the five-years-younger daughter of friends of my parents and had always looked up to me, always wanted everything I had. But most of all, Fridolin. She had gotten her own Fridolin when she was four years old, but after my death, she would have two, hers and the original one.

Martina would inherit all the stories I had written over the years. She had always been one of my biggest supporters when it came to my writing. My stone collection would go to my sister. She was like me—couldn't walk the shore of any beach without her eyes glued to the ground, looking for treasures to take back home.

We had done a few beach vacations together in the past, and it had always been the same picture. On the first day, we would go to the beach, only the pockets of our jackets available to hold stones and shells. None of us wanted to look ridiculous and walk with a bag in hand along the shore. We weren't *that* crazy. Latest by day three we realized, we were *that* crazy and each of us took a bag to the beach. The bags expanded in size toward the end of our vacation until on our last day, on a vacation in Denmark, we used one of the dog leashes to haul a huge boulder, tunneled out by the sea, from the beach back to our car. My sister still had that monstrosity sitting in her living room years later. If anyone would appreciate my stones, it would be her.

Mugs, books, and paintings were promised to several friends, and last, my jewelry would go to Silke, my best friend since middle school.

Silke and I met in fifth grade. At first, we were only classmates, but around sixth grade we became inseparable. The reason why we picked each other as best friends was simple.

"The others were either stupid or didn't want to be friends with us." Silke wasn't shy to explain, but whether she was right or wrong, we fit perfectly together. In German, there's a phrase for that: *Wie Arsch auf Eimer*. We fit together like *ass on bucket*. We sat together in school (as far as teachers let us), sat beside each other on the school bus, met every day after school—wherever one of us went, the other one wasn't far behind. We took care of each other.

First, it was Silke's turn to take care of me. I was a small kid, extremely skinny, big belly, hunched shoulders, yellowish teeth from all the medications I had to take, chronically ill, and therefore the perfect target for bullying. Only problem: no one dared to bully me because of Silke.

Silke has always been very fit and strong. She rode horses during school. Later she would finish the Berlin marathon of 2011 as the fastest German woman; she became a four-time German champion in different running events. And the same determination she would have during her running career, she already possessed as a teen. Determined to do anything she thought was right.

She once chased a group of older boys away, running after them, raised fists, ready to punch them, because they were threatening to throw firecrackers at us, which I was terrified of. When her boyfriend questioned our friendship, she kicked him out of the house, closed the door in his face, and turned off the front porch light, leaving him in the dark. He never got a chance to ask why his relationship with her was history. Silke 100 percent had my back, same as I. When we got older and went to parties, and she got drunk, it was my turn to take care of her. In Germany, you are allowed to drink beer and wine at the age of sixteen, and everyone did, except me. Already then, I had a beginning liver cirrhosis and therefore was always sober when my best friend wasn't.

After parties, drunk or not, we went home together. Sometimes I slept at her place, sometimes she at my place, but always together. Always. Together.

When I was done writing my will, I picked up the phone to call her.

"Hey." Silke answered on the third ring. "What's up? How are you feeling?"

"Hey," I replied, "feeling good, but I'm calling because I have a question. A little out-of-the-ordinary question. You ready?"

"Sure . . ." she said, though it sounded more like a question.

"I just wrote my will," I explained. "Wrote down who will get what if I die. Like who will get my drawings, who will get my stone collection, these kind of things."

A hesitant "okay" came from the other side of the line, but I didn't pay much attention to it. I wanted to get this over with. Get an answer and call the next person on my list.

"I wanted to ask you if there's anything you would like to inherit from me. Anything I don't even know of that reminds you of me. Like a mug, or one of the pictures I have hanging on my walls, anything."

There was a moment of silence. As expected, this was not the ordinary question your friend would ask, and especially not over the phone without warning. I had spent the last two hours thinking about death, my death to be accurate, but Silke was not ready to do the same.

"I don't want you to die." Her voice faltered, then: "Period."

"Well . . ." I suppressed a laugh. "I don't want to die either, but just in case, is there anything you want to inherit from me?"

"This is crazy, you know?" Silke's voice went up an octave. "I understand why you are asking this, I get it, but still, no. Dying is not an option. I don't want one of your coffee mugs, I have my own coffee mugs." Before I could interrupt, she softened with, "I want your phone calls, your letters, postcards—all of that—but not a stupid mug."

I smiled, and it was genuine. "How about my jewelry?"

There was yet another moment of silence, then a theatrical sigh.

"Okay, your jewelry, happy now?" I could almost see her impatiently brushing her long, brown, curly hair out of her face. "Can we talk about something else now? Anything that's not death related?"

Silke never liked to talk about death. I found a strange kind of comfort in it, though. But I had tortured her enough.

"You know I still have the street sign we stole one night. You remember?"

"God, yeah." I could hear she relaxed a little. "You almost freaked out because there was a snail stuck to it and you touched it, without knowing what it was."

I remembered. I screamed so loud, I was surprised we weren't caught.

"You will get that too," I said with a smile in my voice. "Together with the jewelry."

"Cool." This time there was a hint of a smile in her voice too.

"I'm sorry I dumped this on you." And I was. "I'm not planning to die, just so you know. I just want to be prepared is all."

"You should come visit again," Silke said instead of offering an answer. "Maybe next weekend? I have time."

"Yes, sounds good. I'll drive to my parents' house anyway and will stop by on the way. You know, I don't feel comfortable driving that much anymore. My car only drives to hospitals and back these days, but . . ."

"Wait a second," Silke said, not caring anymore what else I had to say. "What about your car? Who will inherit that one?"

And just like that, my black VW Golf 4 became the running joke of my last will because everyone, following Silke's example, *everyone* eventually asked me what I planned to do with it. It was by far the most popular item on my parting gifts list and, in some sense, also the safest. Safe because all the other things on my list presented memories of mine. Every stone I owned was connected to the memory of a vacation. My stuffed seal animal represented my childhood. Every story of mine was a part of me, whereas my car was mostly just that: a car. Everyone could imagine themselves driving in my car, but none of my friends wanted to imagine themselves drinking out of my favorite coffee mug because I wasn't around anymore to drink from it myself. The car was less personal, or at least that's how I interpreted it.

I kept it a secret, but I knew from the moment I taped the wedding car postcard onto the cover of my last will who would get my car. It was the one person who drove me around in it whenever I had to go somewhere and didn't feel well enough to drive myself. A visit to the supermarket, to pick up dog food from the pet store, medications from the pharmacy, or a late-night visit to the hospital—my one and only Aria. Who, by the way, had also asked for it and nothing else.

But in the end, it was exactly that: everyone's *nothing else* that filled my last will with the love I felt for my family and friends. Every *nothing else* had a memory attached to it, and by giving it to the person I had experienced the memory with, that memory would live on. Nothing else and nothing less.

Aria:

- My black Golf 4. You are welcome!

- My *Landliebe* glass. (*Landliebe* is a dairy manufacturer in Germany. In 2001, *Landliebe* offered everyone a cute, flower-printed glass if you sent in a certain number of the German equivalent of box tops. I was one box top short, but I still sent mine in, asking to get a glass nonetheless—and I did. Until today the glass is standing in my kitchen cabinet. Cute as ever.)

- All my crime books and my silver bookmark. Even though Aria never needs a bookmark—she reads that fast.

Silke:

- All my jewelry, especially my half of our friendship ring, and the earring I made from the feathers of Silke's parakeet.

- My Moqui marbles. Moqui marbles are believed to be the most energetic stones on earth and the only stones that come in genders. The rugged one is the male stone, the smooth one the female. I have one of each, lying on my nightstand. They're supposed to bring luck—I guess we will see.

Lydia:

- My Fridolin because Lydia is the only one who understands how important he is.

- The dinosaur egg I found in Italy while on a vacation with her family. It's a stone that truly looks like a dino egg. We tried to make it hatch during our vacation, but as of now, nothing has come out of it.

My Family:

- The Bobby Car my grandpa gave me for Christmas should go to Tina. The only condition: she must have at least one child.

- The golden ring with my mom's initials should go back to her. I know she believes I cursed it because she can't wear it anymore without getting a rash, but I'm sure the curse will be broken once I'm gone.

- The three saint kings I made right before Christmas in 2001, when I still believed my transplant would be near, should also go to my mom. She wanted them from the moment she saw them.

- My scrapbook photo albums should all go to my dad. He will know what to do with them. How to preserve all the happy memories I made in my life.

Shortly after I prepared myself for death, Aria prepared herself for an internship in Belgium. She'd be gone for ten weeks, and I realized I didn't feel fit enough to be home alone, alone without help. I couldn't do grocery shopping by myself anymore. Carrying a gallon of milk up the stairs to our apartment? Impossible. Doing laundry, feeding the dog, walking the dog, cooking dinner, cleaning the house, taking care of my health—beyond impossible. Even my stubbornness wasn't strong enough to overcome that many obstacles.

On February 10, my mom came to pick me up and drove with me to their place. I would spend the next ten weeks with my parents. Of course, I didn't want to live for ten weeks with my parents again. I wanted to be independent from them. It was already hard enough not being independent from my disease anymore, and now I had to deal with unappreciated parental care and advice.

"Enjoy the food," Aria advised before we parted. "Enjoy not having to do anything and meet up with your friends. Ten weeks is not that long, and you can always call or write me."

Turned out, she was right. The first month at my parents' place flew by in a blink of an eye. I kept myself busy with long walks in their forest, meeting friends, and on March 17, I celebrated my twenty-third birthday with many of my old high school friends—Silke included, of course.

It was a wonderful day. A normal day. We all just sat around my parents' dining table in the sunroom, eating cake, drinking tea and coffee, talking, laughing, and joking about old times. My transplant, my current situation, the reason why I lived with my parents right now, had oxygen under my nose, and was coughing more than usual didn't come up. We all pretended it was a normal twenty-third birthday, and I enjoyed pretending to have no worries in the world. It was my last day feeling normal. My last day feeling healthy.

Only one day later, everything changed.

10

Urgent

On my second day as a twenty-three-year-old, I had difficulty breathing. I turned up my oxygen concentrator to blow even more oxygen up my nose. I felt tired, even too tired to eat, and experienced lung bleeding for the first time in my life.

It happened when I went to bed that day. I was just lying down, still searching for the most comfortable position on my pillow, when it suddenly started to bubble in the back of my throat.

I immediately sat back up, started to cough, and there it was: fresh blood. As if someone had stabbed me in the lungs and turned me upside down to let it drop out.

I was concerned—bleeding lungs were never a good sign—but I also knew from other CF patients that it wasn't a reason to freak out over. No need to call an ambulance or a priest. Unless it wouldn't stop. If it wouldn't stop, I would be in deep shit. Internal bleeding from the lungs, esophagus varices, or wherever from could be fatal within minutes. But it did stop. After about five minutes, the bubbling in my throat subsided and I was able to lie down again, only this time very carefully.

From that day on, lung bleeding was looming over my head every night I went to sleep. Most of the time only the fear of it; other times the actual bleeding as well. My lungs were that damaged—I couldn't just lie down anymore and go to sleep. Every night I had to slowly lower myself toward the mattress, one inch at a time, careful not to pop any of my small blood vessels and cause bleeding again.

It sucked.

When I was back in Hannover for another checkup appointment three days later, my doctors were shocked when they saw me. After I had my blood drawn and my lung function taken, the doctor drew a brutally clear picture for me and my sister, who had come with me that day, to make us understand where I was standing at:

"Severely underweight, worsened lung function, increased need for oxygen, not to forget the existing liver cirrhosis. If you want to stay listed for an organ transplant"—she looked me straight in the eyes—"you have to gain weight, build up some muscles, and . . ." She looked at my sister and sighed. "Honestly, we need to reach an acute overall improvement or consider a high urgency listing to prevent failure."

Failure, better known as death, I added. How could it get that bad in such a short time? On my birthday I still felt great, and now we had to achieve an acute improvement for me not to die. How?

"What exactly do you mean by high urgency listing?" Tina asked, way quicker with digesting the news than I.

"Right, let me explain." My doctor straightened up in her seat, happy to talk facts again instead of emotions. "High urgency listing means exactly that: to be listed with a higher urgency," she explained. "Inka could get listed under a higher urgency because she might not be able to survive the length of the normal waiting time. In plain words, she will be placed at the top of the waiting list. If there are organs available, she will be considered first as a recipient because of the urgency of her situation."

In the US, patients who need a lung transplant receive a so-called lung allocation score. The lung allocation score determines the patient's priority for receiving a lung transplant when a donor lung becomes available, also based on the patient's health. A very sick patient would get a higher score and be considered first when a donor lung comes available. Like Europe's high urgency listing.

It sounded perfect.

"So then let's do that," I chimed in. I wanted to bounce off my chair. "If a high urgency listing shortens my wait time, I'm all for it." Duh!

But it wasn't as easy as it sounded. (Is anything?)

"First," my doctor said, "we would have to get approval to list you as high urgency. We would have to do some more tests, present your results to a committee, and the committee would then decide if our request for a high urgency listing is granted or not. If it's granted"—she stopped me before I could yell again *Let's do it*—"you'd have to wait the rest of your wait time in the hospital."

"No waiting at home?" my sister asked, her eyebrows squished together.

"No waiting at home," the doctor confirmed. "Once listed high urgency, you have to stay in the hospital until your transplant."

"And how long is the approximate wait time on the high urgency list?"

This time, it was my sister who asked the question about waiting time, not me. I knew better than that. I didn't want to have anything to do with *approximate* waiting time anymore. It was the same shit as with my normal wait time. No one knew how long I would have to wait, high urgency or not.

"I don't want to know," I wanted to say, about to hold up my hand to stop anything that was coming at me, but my doctor had already answered the question.

"Three weeks," she said. "But it can also take a day or six months. No one knows. Only one thing is certain: Inka will be first in line once organs are available."

It was a tough visit that day. Reality had punched me in the face, and death was waiting around the corner to pick up what was left of me. My lung function was at 25 percent, which meant that my lungs had less capacity than two cans of soda. My weight had dropped by five more pounds to eighty-three pounds. If I lost three more pounds, I would be removed from the waiting list and left to die. Organs were simply too rare to waste on a patient who most likely wouldn't survive the transplant itself. I wondered how my parents would digest the news and if they would feel as numb as me.

After our visit, we sat downstairs again at Hannover's shopping street, trying to digest what we had learned . . . and our lunch. I was again peeling off the pineapple from under the cheese of my Hawaii toast. I threw it into the trash can beside me and then looked over to my sister.

"Why don't you order a toast with cheese if you don't like the pineapple?" she asked with a full mouth.

I shrugged. "This sucks."

We both knew I was not talking about my violated Hawaii toast.

"So, I guess high urgency is not an option for you?" my sister asked, getting straight to the point.

"Can you imagine my mood if I have to wait in the hospital and it'll take months, rather than weeks, before I get transplanted?"

"I really try not to, but I understand what you mean. Mom will suffocate you with a pillow before you get organs."

I nodded. She probably would. Even now, waiting at home with all the comforts one could hope for, I was often insufferable. I was angry, impatient, ungrateful, constantly annoyed, agitated, and scared. And whatever I felt, I shared with everyone around me.

When I was ten years old, the varices in my esophagus burst and I almost died of internal bleeding. The first night in the hospital, the nurse came in to bring me another blood transfusion and I was furious. How could she have the audacity to wake me up in the middle of the night when I already wasn't feeling good? Why couldn't she come later? Or, even better, not at all? I was angry all the time and nasty to everyone: doctors, nurses, my mom included. On the second day, she left my room to cry in the hall and to apologize to the nurses for my disrespectful behavior. But the nurses didn't need an apology. They understood.

"She is fighting for her life," one of them explained to my mom. "She is not ungrateful; she is in battel mode. She will be grateful again when she wins."

And that's exactly what was happening right now. I was fighting for my life with everything I had. With every angry emotion I could come up with. But to know why I behaved like I did didn't change the fact that I couldn't wait for my transplant inside a hospital for an unaccounted amount of time. I had to wait at home. Even if the wait time would be longer. My sanity, the sanity of everyone around me—especially my mom, who would be always by my side—depended on it. Or I swear to God, she truly would suffocate me with my own pillow or strangle me with my bedsheet. We were all just human, and I was very aware of our limitations.

My sister concluded, "So . . . rehabilitation then."

The only other option I had left to save my life.

"I guess," I confirmed. I had never done rehabilitation before, but considering the circumstances, I had to give it a try. During rehab I would get tons of physiotherapy, my diabetes would once more be readjusted, I'd work on building up muscles to gain back some weight, and do another IV therapy to clean out my lungs. And hopefully get a few percent of lung function back.

I quickly decided I wanted to do my rehab up north, along one of the beaches of the North Sea, maybe Norddeich, Harlesiel, or even Langeoog, where my dad had spent most of his childhood vacations. Any of them would be great. Ocean, salty air, crashing waves, beach sand between my toes, and maybe even a small bag slung over my shoulder to collect treasures. If everything else hadn't been so devastating, I might have even been excited.

The next day, my mom was constantly on the phone trying to get my rehab approved and scheduled. In the meantime, my dad cheered me up by doing anything for me. Preparing a delicious lunch, plugging a good movie into the DVD player, and motivating me to take one last walk with my dog around the neighborhood. My last walk, because later my sister stopped by and took my dog with her.

It had been a decision of the whole family, me included, but it didn't make it any easier letting her go. I knew Fenja was way better off at my sister's place. Most of the day outside, together with my sister's dog, going on long walks, or on horseback-riding excursions. I had barely enough strength left to take her around the block but still . . . when my sister left, my dog in tow, I hit rock bottom. And there was only one person I felt comfortable turning to.

Dear Ingo,

I'm so sad, so down, so broken into a million pieces! Since today I'm without my dog. Fenja will live with Tina until further notice. It was the right decision, for sure, but it still feels as if my life is nothing but a pile of fragments. As if it isn't even my life anymore.

Did you feel the same the sicker you got? As if you were dissolving into nothingness between countless hospital visits and bad news?

I have to go to rehabilitation within the next few days. To rehab, dear God. It sounds as if I'm sick or something. When you wrote me your letter, you'd also been in rehab, right? Or was it at a hospital? I don't remember. But I do remember a week later, you were dead. Well, at least my mom will accompany me, hold my hand, as if I'm on my deathbed already.

Don't worry, though, I don't think I'm dying quite yet, but death did come a huge step closer. I can't just relax anymore, let the doctors talk and wait for my miracle to happen. Now I really have to pull myself together and fight. Drink nasty calorie drinks to gain weight, check my blood sugar all the time, and start moving my body again. If I lose more weight, more muscles, they'll take me off the waiting list and won't transplant me. Can you imagine? Tables and numbers

> decide if I get a second chance or not. A doctor can decide to seal my death sentence, just because he or she thinks I won't survive the transplant as skinny as I am. Gods in white. Maybe there is some truth to it after all.
>
> I don't know where to put my despair and how to cope with the nonstop feeling of me-against-the-world, but one thing I'm telling you, I won't give up! I won't die! Fuck that! — Your wanting-to-show-everyone-the-middle-finger niece

After a whole day on the phone, my mom got the approval for my rehab from the health insurance in record time. And only twenty-four hours later, we had it in writing. I was allowed to spend six to eight weeks in a rehab center of my choice. It was a miracle. For the first time in forever, I was excited. I felt like I was about to go on a mini vacation, humming a constant tune, laughing out loud at the weirdest moments and getting on my mom's nerves. I was so looking forward to new surroundings. A new daily routine. New people to talk to. Finally, an escape from the days at my parents' house that stretched like gum. Always the same, never-ending, only their flavor fading the more I chewed. But with rehab in sight, I could already see myself walking along the beach, my mom by my side, picking up shells, breathing in the salty ocean air, then physiotherapy, building up muscles until I was again the fittest patient they had ever seen. I was so ready. Ready to thrive.

But life had to be a bitch.

The first rehab center my mom called had empty beds, but all the other CF patients at that facility didn't have the bacteria called pseudomonas in their lungs. I, however, did.

(Of *course* I did.)

Pseudomonas is not dangerous, but for CF patients, it can be. Under no circumstances would anyone allow me to be mixed with CF patients who were pseudomonas-free. I couldn't come, not until all the other patients had finished their rehab three weeks from now.

But I didn't have that time.

Another two rehab centers had the same story—having pseudomonas-free patients—and weren't able to accept me. The last two centers my mom called were not even close to the North Sea, but we were getting desperate. Someone had to take me. Someone had to help me get back on my feet—sand between my toes or not. But also, the last two rehab centers couldn't accept me. They were fully booked.

Nobody was able to accept me as their patient. Nobody was able to help me survive and make it to my transplant. Fucking nobody.

I felt like roadkill. Being hit, lying on the side of the highway, barely breathing, barely alive, while everyone else zoomed by because no one cared, no one had time to care, and no one had an empty seat in their car. It was a feeling of utter helplessness. Like the feeling when the doctor didn't want to give me the right dosage of antibiotics when I was hospitalized as a teen; same as then, I couldn't do anything to change the situation I was in. I couldn't force any rehabilitation center to take me. I couldn't argue, negotiate, or bribe. The system was fully booked and therefore failing me. An experience I never had before. Growing up, it had never happened that there was no capacity to help me. It had never happened that a hospital was too full to help save my life. This was Germany, for Christ's sake. Not a third-world country. And still, I was left alone. Help wouldn't come any time soon.

I wanted to make myself small—so small that I'd just fall in between the cracks of the floor and be gone for good.

But my stubbornness wouldn't let me.

Instead, I got pissed. I didn't allow myself to feel discouraged or tempted to give up as my mom feared. I was angry. Oh, so angry. If no one was ready to help me survive, fuck it, I'd do it myself. Anything rehab would do, I could do too. Eating more—done. Building up muscles, dragging myself every day to the gym to do something—done. Showing everyone the middle finger and taking care of my own survival—done too.

While my mom secretly cried because she couldn't do anything to help her daughter get a fair chance of survival, I raised my middle fingers to the world. One thing was for sure: I would not die just because the rehab centers wouldn't take me. Not in a million years.

11

Memories

I was still ready to fight the world all by myself the next morning, still holding my middle finger up for everyone to see, still angry that there wasn't a single rehab room available . . . until the phone rang and we finally got good news.

Even though it had felt like no one cared to fight for me, my transplant team in Hannover had and they had found a place for me. I was beyond grateful. Not in a rehab center—they truly were all fully booked—but a place in their hospital. I would do everything I had planned to do at rehab, only now at the hospital: IV therapy, everyday physiotherapy, diabetes training once again, and high-calorie food intake. I wouldn't get to sink my toes into beach sand or feel the waves lick at my feet, but that was okay. If ugly Hannover was ready to lend me a hand, I was ready to take it. We immediately packed our things and left to claim my spot.

My hospital-based rehab started on March 27. Three-times-a-day antibiotic infusion, everyday physiotherapy, stretching, massages, and training to build up muscle, but that wasn't all Hannover had in mind. They also wanted me to get a PEG.

"A PEG?" I shook my head. It was the first time my doctor mentioned it to me.

"It's not a big deal," he immediately reassured me. "It's a small procedure where a feeding tube is inserted through a small incision into your upper abdomen. The tube is then connected to your stomach, and you can receive extra nutrition overnight. You won't even feel it. You will be fed while you sleep and will be able to gain weight much faster."

He looked at me like a salesperson offering the deal of a lifetime.

I was not convinced.

"How do you know that I won't even feel it?" I crossed my arms, and the doctor stole a glance at my mom. "And how do you know the whole procedure is not a big deal? Did you ever get a PEG?"

His salesperson's smile crumbled.

"No, I haven't," he confessed. "But the procedure is short. It only takes about twenty minutes to place a PEG. Most patients are very happy with their PEG, and all of them gain weight. All of them."

"I will gain weight by myself," I said. "I've always been a good eater. I don't want a PEG. At least not yet."

"Please think about it," my doctor said and stood up to leave. When the door closed behind him, my mom turned to face me.

"Why?" she said, gazing upward, as if God could help her put sense into her daughter's mind. "Why always the more difficult route? Why not for once agree to what the doctor suggests and be done with it?"

"First," I said, looking straight into her narrowing eyes, "because I was raised to question every doctor I will ever encounter in my life."

My mother couldn't do anything else but nod in agreement. Indeed, that was how I was raised. For better, for worse.

"And second," I said, "because I don't want to wake up every morning feeling stuffed because they pumped me with calorie drinks during the night and have my appetite for breakfast ruined. I love to eat. If I feel stuffed, I want it to be because I ate too much delicious food and not because someone filled my stomach while I was asleep."

My mom held my stare, looked for something to say to prove me wrong, but eventually just said, "Fair enough."

Of course she wanted me to get a PEG. I was her daughter; she was ready to try anything to save my life. Especially after we had come so close to getting no help at all, she was grateful for any. But on the other hand, she was as food-driven as I and understood how I wanted to eat and enjoy every calorie I had to gain, and not have them forced into me.

"Hawaii toast then?" my mom asked instead of giving me another lecture, and I agreed. I didn't want a PEG; I had to eat as much as I could. And there was no better time than to start right now.

"And maybe afterward some cake," I added as a sign of my goodwill, gathered my things, and followed my mom down to the shopping street. It was way more fun gaining weight this way than while sleeping at night. My mom agreed while she ordered a huge piece of cake for herself as well.

I stayed for two weeks in the hospital. It was boring as hell, even with cake and Hawaii toast in the afternoons, but my health improved. I gained 500ml of lung capacity, my weight increased by one and a half pounds, I was able to walk upstairs again, ride the stationary bicycle, and play catch with my mom in the hospital garden on the weekends, when there was no other entertainment available.

But we also did other stuff. Forbidden stuff. Forbidden by the hospital, my doctors, my nurses, everyone. We left the hospital and drove to my aunt's place, Renate, thirty minutes away, where I showered every other day. I hated the showers at the hospital. They were old, and I never felt clean after using them. Taking a shower at my aunt's place felt so much better. It always felt like a moment of normality standing in her clean bathroom, using a fluffy towel, smelling fancy shampoo, and using appliances that weren't made from metal but white ceramic. As if I were normal and not sickling away.

When Easter came around, we pushed our limit even farther and drove to the Hannover Zoo. I wasn't a huge zoo fan, but there we could walk around, take a break at a café whenever I needed one, enjoy flowers and greenery, and walk beside happy children running around and having a blast. Joy—you didn't get to see that inside the Hannover Medical School.

We spent all afternoon at the zoo. Walked around the whole compound, me carrying oxygen slung over my shoulder, stopping at every other café to eat non-hospital food, watching families walk by, enjoying a normal day at the zoo, same as us. It was such a needed break from everything going on in my life. As if death had taken a break too and was not chasing me that afternoon.

When we came back to the hospital, we both had a huge smile on our faces, until one of my nurses stopped us in the hall, demanding to know:

"Where have you been? We've been calling your name over the intercom all afternoon. We needed you in your room to place a new IV access."

Dang.

I immediately felt guilty and didn't know what to say. My mom, not so much.

"Oh," she said, seemingly shocked by what we had missed, "we were sitting outside in the hospital garden all afternoon. I guess we couldn't hear the intercom over there. So sorry."

The venous access was placed once I was back in my room. No harm done. Of course, we knew from the beginning leaving the hospital grounds was risky. If anything happened to me outside of the hospital—a car accident, attack of a tiger, anything—the insurances would go berserk trying to figure out who was responsible. But still, it was worth the risk. This could be the last time I had in my life. I couldn't just sit inside the hospital and let that time waste away. I had to use it somehow, and thanks to my mom, who saw it the same way I did, we had. Our time at the zoo, the moments we had shared, the many laughs and coffees—no one could take these memories from us. And that's what it was all about, memories. As many memories as possible that made life count.

At the beginning of April, I was back home. Revived and already looking forward to my next mini vacation. Since my hospital rehab had been billed as a normal hospital stay, I still had the insurance-approved rehab available to utilize and my mom had finally scheduled a rehab place, a real one this time. And not only any rehab place. This one was in St. Peter-Ording, right on the coast of the North Sea.

St. Peter-Ording looks like most northern beach vacation towns. Ice cream carts, fresh-seafood-on-a-bun stands everywhere, same as souvenir shops. The beach, on the other hand, was special in St. Peter-Ording, as they didn't have the usual narrow line of sand, but rather a half-mile-wide, seven-mile-long sanded coastline. At some places one could even drive with the car along the beach or do land sailing. I couldn't wait to go. I could already see myself walking along the beach, collecting stones and shells, a salty taste on my lips, and a fresh shrimp sandwich in my hand. But as always, life had to be a bitch. On my second day back home from my rehab at the hospital, I woke up in the morning with a crazy headache and nausea.

Okay, I thought. *This is nothing. Just some headache, it'll go away, all good.*

I made myself sit through breakfast and forced a few bites of toast down my throat, but soon I had to lie down again. The constant throbbing left me downright exhausted. Was my nausea simply nausea, or was it a result of the skull-breaking headache?

My mom brought me some headache pills, which I swallowed as quickly as possible, not to barf them right back up again, and went back to sleep. I knew something was wrong, majorly wrong, but I didn't want to believe it. I had just spent two weeks at the hospital. Two weeks of IVs and therapy, two weeks of being poked, examined, and evaluated. There was no way I could be sick again. There was no way I would *accept* being sick again. I only needed a few more hours of sleep. Then the headache would be gone, and everything would be great.

Utter bullshit, of course, but I still wanted to believe it.

My mom woke me a couple of hours later, and I felt even worse. My headache was so bad, I wasn't able to sit up without fearing my head might explode.

"Do you want another Advil?" My mom sat at the side of my bed, stroking my hair; worry was written all over her face. Like me, she couldn't believe this was happening, and so shortly after my hospital stay.

But my dad cut to the chase.

"She doesn't need Advil," he said, leaving the doorframe behind he had just been leaning against, giving my mom a curt nod. "She needs to go to the hospital. Immediately. I'll get the car. You get her a jacket. Let's go."

My dad parked the car right in front of our door while my mom helped me to put a jacket, socks, and shoes on. I couldn't lift my head due to the pain and then realized I wouldn't be able to sit in the car either.

"I can't sit," I told my mom while she tightened my shoelaces. "I need to lie down in the car. I don't know how, but I can't sit. My head . . ." My voice trembled. I didn't really know what to say. This was bad. Not only because I had just come back home from two weeks of intensive hospital care, but because I had no idea what was going on. It wasn't my lungs or my liver causing this much pain, so what the hell was?

My dad heard me and went to crank the co-pilot seat as far back as possible. I wouldn't be lying down, but I wouldn't be sitting either. Hopefully good enough for our fifteen-minute drive to the hospital.

He helped me get in the car, buckled my seatbelt for me, and told my mom to call him as soon as I was taken care of. As always, my dad stayed home. If he had to, he would have been by my side, but it was better for everyone if he stayed home and let my mom handle the rest.

My mom knew her way around an emergency room. She knew how to address doctors, how to persuade nurses to get her a cup of coffee, and how not to faint when it came to needles, body fluids, and invasive procedures. My dad wouldn't have fainted either, but he would have felt just wrong. The doctor's words would have sounded like Chinese to him. He wouldn't have known if it was okay to drink coffee or where to ask for some, and after seeing needles being poked into his daughter's arms, he wouldn't even have known if he wanted coffee at all. His help and support would be needed once the emergency was taken care of. He'd give hope to my mom if she'd come home with bad news, and he'd do anything to cheer me up while I had to stay in the hospital. This was how it had always been and how our family worked best. Everyone had their role to stick to. I was the sick one, my mom took care of me, my dad took care of everything else, and my sister would only be called in if shit hit the fan.

Once during the drive to the hospital, my mom had to stop at the side of the road because I thought I had to throw up. False alarm.

We were silent for most of the drive. Me concentrating on my breathing, trying not to throw up or lose it completely because I was that scared, and my mom concentrating on the road and trying to keep her motherly worries bottled up as well. But when we drove onto the full parking lot of the hospital, I couldn't keep it together any longer. I was drenched in sweat, I felt terrible and somehow . . . like dying?

"Mom, I'm losing it," I said, eyes closed, holding on to what was left of me. "I need to get to the hospital. Right now."

My eyes were still closed, but I could almost sense my mom going pale, tightening her grip on the steering wheel. Then I actually feel her making a sharp turn, wheels squealing on the asphalt.

"What?" My eyes flew wide open.

"I'll get you there," my mom answered without looking at me. All her attention was at the entrance of the hospital, where we were heading right now, where I had to be.

She wasn't allowed to drive right to the entrance of the hospital, taxis only, but she didn't hesitate taking the last turn. Not even when she realized she was driving against the traffic.

The car came to an abrupt halt right beside the sliding doors of the hospital. My mom pulled the handbrakes with unnecessary force, leaving a ratcheting sound behind. She jumped out of the car and ran inside the hospital. A security guard in a bluish-gray uniform yelled after her, but the doors had already closed behind her.

He glanced in my direction, but my appearance made it obvious I wasn't the right one to talk to. For a second, it looked like he would run after my mom inside the hospital, but then he just crossed his arms in a wide stance and waited for her to come back to get a piece of his mind.

I didn't care. I only wanted to get inside the hospital. Inside their ER. A doctor by my side who made sure I wouldn't die because that's how I felt. I felt like my body was about to just stop working. Without me even knowing why. I didn't know what had caused this. I didn't know what was wrong and therefore felt helpless to do anything to prevent it.

The only thing I could do was shove some glucose tablets into my mouth and suck on them. My sweating didn't feel like too low blood sugar, but who knew. If it truly was too low blood sugar, I could do something about it. If not, it wouldn't hurt.

I was on my third glucose tablet, beads of sweat still dripping off my lip and forehead, when the sliding doors of the hospital opened again and my mom came out, followed by a nurse pushing a wheelchair.

The security guard immediately jumped into action, making space for them as if they had to push their way through a mob of people. If I hadn't felt like dying, I might have laughed at the sight.

My mom opened my door and helped me get into the wheelchair. She didn't say a word. She looked as determined as I felt to get me near a doctor, any doctor, and to safety. The nurse looked the same. Furrowed brows and an alert gaze on her face.

With a groan of pain, I fell into the chair. My head felt as if it might roll off my shoulders and down the sidewalk, but thank God it didn't. The nurse turned me around and rushed back inside the hospital; my feet weren't even placed on the footrests yet. My mom yelled something after me that sounded like: "I'll be right back. I need to park the car."

I was through the sliding doors, greeted by a doctor who helped me lie down on a hospital bed already waiting for me.

My head touched the pillow, a blanket was pulled over me, and I was wheeled to the ER, the doctor walking alongside me while talking, but I didn't listen. I had only room for one thought, and one thought only: I was safe. I wouldn't die in the passenger seat of my mom's car, without even knowing why. I was finally safe. I was so relieved; if I would've had the strength, I would have cried.

My ER doctor figured out pretty quickly what was wrong with me. It wasn't too low blood sugar; it wasn't an acute case of dying. It was a simple stomach virus. A virus I had picked up in Hannover, during my so-called rehabilitation. Again, I would have cried if I could have.

"But how can a simple stomach virus make her that sick?" My mom asked exactly what I was asking myself. *How?*

"Well . . ." The doctor pulled one of the puke-green plastic ER chairs closer and sat down. "She is very weak to begin with. Her body has probably no resources anymore to fight a simple virus beside everything else that's going on."

"And what do we do now?" My mom had already digested the fact that I was in deep shit and was ready to roll up her sleeves, get to work, and get better. Me? Not so much. I had just worked my ass off for two weeks to get back on my feet. I had done everything I could to gain back some weight, to be active again, to build up muscles, and now it turned out to be all for nothing because of a stomach virus? Maybe I couldn't cry because crying was not enough to express how I felt.

I looked at my mom, trying to communicate to her without saying a word that I wouldn't roll up my sleeves again and fight for my life—fuck that—but she didn't look at me. She only looked at the doctor who was about to deliver the final blow.

"There's not much we can do at this point," he said, slowly getting off his chair, ready to leave to see another patient. "A virus can't be fought with antibiotics or any other medication. All we can do is wait and support Inka's body in fighting it by itself."

"Supporting it how?" Once again, my mom.

"We will give her IV fluids, pain medication as needed, and hopefully soon she'll be able to eat again and get back to her feet."

"What if she won't be able to eat any time soon? She can't afford to lose more weight. If she loses more weight, she'll be taken off the transplant list."

"In that case, we might consider more drastic measures, like, for example . . ."

"A PEG?" I asked, my hand jerking forward as if I were reaching for the last straw, my gaze darting back and forth between my mom and my doctor. I needed something to hold on to, anything—even a PEG would do just to keep me afloat.

For the first time, the doctor turned his attention to me and nodded. "Yes," he said, "we might consider a PEG."

"Can I get one right now? A PEG, I mean." I could barely lie still anymore. "I haven't eaten anything since this morning. I'm fasting. There is no reason to wait." If the doctor would have pointed me in the right direction, I would have jumped out of bed and ran to the operating room myself, but both the doctor and my mom just looked at me as if I had lost my mind.

"You want a PEG?" my mom asked in disbelief. "Are you sure? Last time we talked about it, you were absolutely against it. Remember? *I don't want to feel stuffed in the morning* and all of that."

"Not anymore," I said angrily. Did no one around me understand how urgent this matter was? Were they all stupid? "I will die if I can't eat. I need a PEG. I need one right now."

My mom and I glowered at each other, both silent, both trying to keep our fear at bay, until my mom turned her attention back to the doctor. She probably thought, *Better seize the moment and get a PEG into that child before she decides otherwise.*

"Is that possible?" she asked.

"No," he said without hesitation. "We already talked to Hannover, and your doctors in Hannover want to wait before we fall back to a solution that will involve surgery. Right now, in the state you're in, the procedure of placing a PEG will only increase the risk of your body not being able to handle everything that's thrown at it. We'll wait a few days. Hopefully by then, you'll feel better and there won't be a need for anything besides rest and high-calorie food."

With that, he excused himself and I couldn't stop the tears from coming anymore.

12

My Second Life

When they moved me from the ER to my new room, I was sure they'd take me downstairs, all the way underground to the cold basement and park my bed right beside the morgue. Instead, I was placed in a bright room where I just lay, thinking of my stomach virus and how it could cost me my life. The morgue would have been fine as well.

My mom spent most of the time on the phone. She talked to my dad, my sister, Martina; the rest of the time, she tried to find something to do. She brought me a pouch of applesauce from the cafeteria downstairs, as well as a bottle of water and some apple juice, and made sure the remote control was near and working.

When the nurse brought my dinner that I wasn't able to eat, Mom gathered up her things, ready to head home.

"I'll see you in the morning?" she asked, not sure herself if she should leave or stay.

I just nodded.

"If there's anything you need, call me." She pointed at my phone lying right next to me on the nightstand and gave me a kiss on my forehead.

Again, I just nodded. I was tired. Exhausted physically and mentally. All I could think was, *I wish I wasn't here. I wish I could be the one saying goodbye to me and being able to drive home for the night.*

I wished for anything but this.

When the door closed behind my mom, I caught that hesitant look on her. I only wanted to do one thing: remove myself from this misery by falling asleep. But my headache was still that bad, especially after I had cried for so long that I couldn't sleep.

I reached over to my nightstand, not grabbing my phone but the call button for my nurse. If I wanted to sleep, I needed pain medication. Strong pain medication.

"I'll bring you some Tylenol. Drops, maybe, not a pill," the nurse said once she arrived, standing beside my bed. She was back out the door before I could even argue with her.

"Tylenol?" I muttered to myself and clenched my teeth, trying to stop another downfall of tears.

I didn't need Tylenol. I didn't wake up in the morning with a hangover; I was struggling to stay alive. Tylenol felt like I was given a toothpick to fight off a hungry lion. I needed something way stronger, but from experience, I knew most nurses simply couldn't distinguish between a chronically ill patient who won't cry for painkillers unless they are truly needed, and a patient who felt close to death because of a pulled toenail. I had to play the game, as always.

When my nurse came back to my room with my Tylenol drops, I didn't argue. I knew what was going to happen if I swallowed the bitter drops and I decided to show her instead of wasting time with long, ignored explanations.

I sat up, swallowed the drops, and immediately barfed them back up. Into the kidney dish the drops had been delivered.

The next time my nurse came in, she brought an IV. She must've talked to my doctor, not wanting to risk having to change my bedsheets if I barfed again.

"This will help," she promised, then hooked me up and started the drip.

And it did.

The medication was that strong. After a few minutes, I couldn't feel my hands and feet anymore, nor my head. Everything went numb. I wasn't worried anymore that I would die. I didn't feel pain or discomfort anymore. I was finally able to sleep and forget. One of the very few grateful moments of my pre-transplant time.

The next day, I already felt a tiny bit better. I still wasn't able to sit up without experiencing a vicious comeback of a headache, but I ate a few pretzels here and there and a few bites of toast my mom had brought up to my room. I was able to drink enough to be taken off the IV fluids too.

I was still worried about my weight, as a few pretzels weren't enough to keep me stable, but I felt somehow in control again. I wasn't completely helpless anymore. I could eat. And I would eat. As much and as often as humanly possible. I would get the lost weight back. I would survive this. Without a PEG.

Yes, only twelve hours after I begged my doctor to place a PEG into my abdomen, right here, right now, I was convinced I could do without. My fear of dying was fading, as well as my willingness to turn to desperate measures. I just had to eat and stubbornly hold on to life. And if I was capable of anything, it was being stubborn. When my mom left to eat lunch at the downstairs cafeteria, I knew what I had to do.

The moment the door closed behind her and I was alone, I carefully sat up—not too much to cause a headache—and reached for the high-calorie drink my mom had left on my nightstand.

Even without a headache and persisting nausea, all the high=calorie drinks I had ever tried were disgusting. The latest one, standing on my nightstand right now, was orange flavor. It came in an eight-ounce cup, lid on top, and tasted a little bit like Gatorade mixed with disgustingness.

I took a deep breath and told myself: *This is what you have to do*. I had to get calories into my body, and I would.

I took off the lid, peeled off the seal, and gulped it down as fast as possible. Trying not to taste anything. Trying to do it in a swift motion before my stomach could alert the press.

Well, it didn't work.

Everything came back up the moment it was down, and because I didn't have a kidney dish nearby, I threw it all back up into the cup it had come from. It fit perfectly. I put the lid back on, put it back on my nightstand, and that was it. *I hope no one tries to steal a sip from that cup.*

No extra calories yet, but I'd try again later. My stomach might have been upset, but I wasn't giving up. I'd get back on my feet if it was the last thing I did.

When my mom came back from lunch and sat down beside my bed, her eyes caught sight of the cup with the high-calorie drink inside.

"Maybe you should try and drink one of these?" She pointed at it.

"I already drank it once," I told her.

It took her a moment to understand and to get up to flush it down the sink.

On my third day, I was able to sit up again without a headache and eat breakfast. I felt invincible. I felt strong. I felt like I had this totally under control. I had probably lost some weight, but I had an appetite, I was eating, I was allowed to order pizza or any other food I desired, and I was back on track. Or at least that's what it felt like. Reality only hit me a few days later, when I was released to go back home.

My mom was downstairs, carrying some of my accumulated stuff to the car. We were going home today. Tomorrow I would have to go back to my daily physiotherapy. I would probably drive a bit on the stationary bicycle, lift a few pathetic-looking weights, and do some stretching. There was no reason for me to just sit and wait for tomorrow to come. I could start moving right now, right here, by carrying the two empty water bottles I still had in my room outside to place them in the cart designated for them.

I felt good doing something. Cleaning up by myself and not letting my mom do everything for me as she had the last few days. But walking with two empty water bottles in my hands was almost too much for me. When I reached my door, I was so exhausted that I had to sit down on one of the benches in the hall, one thankfully right in front of my room.

I could see the cart for the empty water bottles. It was maybe twenty feet away. A few steps, and I'd be there, but I couldn't.

"Can I help you?" A nurse was looking down at me while I hugged my two empty bottles.

"No," I said. "I just need a moment." My legs felt weak and were shaking with fatigue. I needed a moment to convince them that they were able to carry me over to the cart and back. They had to, or I'd army crawl. Dammit, I'd get there.

She nodded and hurried on to assist the next patient who had pressed their call button for help as I stood up again.

I made it to the cart and back to my room, but I was exhausted and shocked by how much effort it took me to walk fifty feet, including two bench breaks. I had felt so great and strong, sitting in my bed, eating like a normal person, but now I realized, the stomach virus had truly left me dangling from a thread.

Throughout all my waiting time, I had never been and would never be as weak and as skinny as I was back then. My weight was seventy-seven pounds, and I found out a bit later that Hannover had paused my listing for an organ transplant during that time. I was still listed but not actively. If there had been an offer for organs during this time, they would have given them to someone else. Not to discourage me, my mom only told me about it later and I was very grateful for that. I had survived my stomach virus and could move on without loss.

It was excruciatingly difficult to get my body back to where it had been before the stomach virus. During my daily physiotherapy, I was constantly ready to crumble to the ground, rest my weary limbs, and sleep for five weeks. Every walk to the restroom at my parents' house felt uphill, and the way back the same. Small things like brushing teeth, putting on clothes, taking a shower—things most people did without even noticing—left me bone-weary. But still, slowly, slowly, one ounce of weight at a time, I recovered and eventually was placed back onto the wait list for my organ transplants. I was relieved to hear that no organs had come available during my recovery time from the stomach virus.

I hadn't missed my maybe one and only chance of a second life due to a virus. Nothing had changed. I was still waiting. Already for seven months. If anyone still believed in the transplant . . . I didn't know. It felt like everyone was so accustomed to me waiting, to me being at home with my parents, to me doing nothing, no one would be surprised or disappointed if my call for donor organs never came. Even to me the idea of *the* call became more and more alien the longer I waited. Could it really happen? Would I truly be transplanted at some point in time? And if not, what would happen then? Could life truly go on without me? My parents' lives? My sister's life? My friends' lives?

The more I thought about my second life, the more I felt like I had to make it. The more the waiting time dragged on, the more I felt like I had to survive, or everything else—and I mean *everything*—would be for nothing. I don't know if it was more a burden or a motivator, but death became less of an option.

April 18, 2002

> Since I have experienced the fear of dying, my life feels unbelievably full again. Like a huge rubber ball. Normally the ball is moderately filled. I just live my life. I have some dreams and hopes. Nothing spectacular. But my wishing ball is now filled with so much more, I'm afraid it might burst before I can start living it. Everything becomes important, beautiful, and meaningful, it almost suffocates me. I can't imagine anything that could make me mad or make me suffer in my new life. Life would be perfect if I would just

be able to breathe. All the things you can do when you can breathe. Jogging, running . . . if in a hurry, then swimming, jumping, dancing—so much power and energy! And once I have lots of energy, I can do even more things. Cooking for a long time, laughing for a long time, staying up for a long time—long, long, long. Okay, for sure every day—life will catch up with me at some point and the ball will shrink again, but right now, it's unbearably full. It feels like so much life is inside of me just waiting to get out.

April 19, 2002

Life's not only gaining on content, but also on meaning. Suddenly everything I still want to experience in life seems so important. The thought, that I might not be able to live it all, seems terrible. Normally I don't value life that high. Once it's over, it's over. I can be happy with the life I had so far, but still, it feels terrible, if that would be it. I already fought too much, developed too many dreams not to make it. The fear of death becomes more and more with every wish I dare to dream. The fear that all my wishes might not come true grows. And the already experienced life shrinks as if I can't imagine a fulfilled life anymore without new organs.

On May 7, on a sunny Tuesday morning, my mom and I packed our bag and drove up north to the coast to St. Peter-Ording, where I would finally start my first rehab. At the exact rehab I was supposed to go before my stomach virus knocked me down, the exact rehab that couldn't accept me earlier due to the pseudomonas virus I had and others didn't. Now, all the other CF patients at St. Peter-Ording would have the same virus I had, and I was free to come, finally. This time, everything was planned perfectly. My mom had rented a small apartment close to the rehab clinic where she could stay for the first week of my rehab. She'd could help me settle in and be close by just in case I needed something. It comforted me to have her so close.

The rehab clinic itself had a single room reserved for me. Up front I had received a list of activities offered to patients when outside of therapy, and I was allowed to use their saltwater pool as often as I felt like.

It all sounded great. The clinic itself looked great too. A huge rectangle building, accented with red bricks and balconies here and there, overall friendly, and bright-looking. Also, the inside was welcoming. More like a grand reception area of a hotel than a hospital. And still, even though I had been looking forward to this day, to my rehab at the Northern Sea, the moment we arrived, all I wanted to do was turn around and go back home. Back to the routine I already knew. I felt too exhausted to settle into a new room. Too tired to learn where I had to go for my meals, and too distraught to listen to anything the nurse told and asked me during my intake interview.

"Can we finish the interview later?" I eventually asked her. "I need to rest a little bit before I can go on."

If the nurse was taken aback by my question, she didn't show.

"Of course." She smiled at me, exchanged one concerned look with my mom, and then arranged for someone to come show me to my room. Only one more question she asked before I was released:

"Before you rest," she said, "I only need to know one thing: Do you want me to apply for four additional weeks of rehab, or rather only do the four weeks you are originally here for?"

My mom and I looked confused.

"Could you repeat that?" my mom asked, glancing at me as if looking for answers, but I didn't have any either. "An additional four weeks of rehab? Following the four we already got approved?"

The nurse nodded. "We encourage every patient who might need more time than four weeks in rehab to immediately apply for an extension the moment they arrive. This way the insurance has enough time to grant you the extension before your first four weeks end, and you can simply stay in your room and continue with your stay uninterrupted. Make sense?"

My mom nodded and looked at me, but under no circumstances was I ready to stay one day longer than I had to. I was too weak to be able to sit through a one-hour interview, so how could anyone expect me to scream "Hurray!" when offered an extended stay at a facility I haven't even gotten to know yet?

I was worried my room would be too far from the dining room. That I would struggle every day to get to breakfast, lunch, and dinner. I was worried about what kind of therapies I would get. If I were strong enough to exercise and still be able to shower at the end of the day. I was way too exhausted to welcome anything new and therefore said no to any extension of my stay.

If the nurse would have asked me one week later, my answer would have been a cheerful yes. After one week of rehab, I was married to my new routine and would have done anything to stay longer. I loved it at rehab. It felt like living in a disease-protected bubble. At rehab, I didn't feel sick, I didn't feel limited or as if my life was on hold. I had things to do at rehab. I had places to be, I had appointments, I had options on what I wanted to do during my free time (things like drawing a picture on a huge silk cloth, or sewing a teddy bear) and, best of all, I got to handle everything by myself. My mom wasn't there to take me to my daily physiotherapy. My mom wasn't the one who reminded me every day when it was time to get ready for walking group. I had to make sure I arrived everywhere on time. I felt like a whole person again, like a grown-up, a person with self-responsibility.

And it felt fuckin' great.

My first three weeks at rehab flew by way too fast. It felt like it had only been a few days when my mom was back to stay the last week with me, like she had the first week of my rehab. She rented the same apartment as before, and we made the best of the last seven days we had.

One afternoon, we walked from the clinic all the way, about two miles, to the shore of the North Sea. I took some pictures of the picturesque stilt houses by the sea, watched land sailors in the distance, and collected a few shells.

Another day we walked to the city center. Cobblestone sidewalks, small, red brick houses leaning against each other, fighting the constant breeze from the sea, fresh seafood sandwiches, souvenir shops, and an ice cream for the way back. And then, on our last day, we did something my dad would have never allowed if I had been healthy and not currently dying: we took my car and drove it on the beach. To be more accurate, *I* took my car and drove it along the beach. It was awesome.

My mom was constantly worried we would get stuck somewhere in the sand, that the tide would come back, make the sea level rise, and then my car would be history.

My dad, though back home, was constantly worried about rust to the car. I could almost hear him saying "Saltwater is death for the car!" every time I drove through a puddle of seawater.

And I wasn't worried at all for once. The music was blaring, salty air rushing through the open windows of the car, seagulls flying overhead—this was another moment I had experienced in life, and death wouldn't be able to take it from me.

June 3, my last happy day of the summer. Because as expected, when I got back home on June 4 and left the protective bubble of rehab, I fell into a deep, dark hole of self-pity, despair, frustration, boredom, and especially the *willingness* to suffer.

13

Happy

The first two weeks back home after rehab felt like Thanksgiving without gravy.

I was inconsolable. Most of the time, I only wanted to sit around and cry. One evening it got so bad that my sister came over and picked me up to spend the weekend at her place. It helped me to get away from my parents for a few nights. It helped me to get away from anything normal that only showed me how normal wasn't possible for me anymore. I was so tired of fighting my decline every day, over and over and over again, without being able to take a break and without being able to see any kind of horizon. There was no promise of how long I still had to suffer. There was no end to all of this, and I struggled to accept it.

After watching me at rock bottom and not being able to pick myself back up again, my mom decided to take matters into her own hands. Or rather, give matters into the hands of a psychologist.

I knew immediately a psychologist wouldn't be able to help me. I had sat through enough lectures to be able to tell salivation for food and salivation for no food apart. Seeing a psychologist would be the latter. Getting all excited, drooling all over the place for no reward at the end. Maybe if said psychologist had the right blood type and was willing to donate some organs I'd get something out of it, but otherwise, no way.

Still, I went. More for my mom than for myself. I didn't do much for others during my waiting time; I was mostly concentrated on myself, but from time to time, it did occur to me how my parents were suffering too. It was not all about me—not all the time at least—and that's why I went.

I went to see my psychologist three times and then gave up. Because my psychologist couldn't help me either. I had to suffer through my waiting time; there was no way around it. I had filled that time with as many activities as I could: photography, writing, crafting, reading, watching TV. There was no magic activity I hadn't tried yet that would make the days feel shorter. Positive thinking? I was way past that. I had nothing left inside of me to think much at all. I felt empty and exhausted, and there was nothing any psychologist in the world could do about it. Time for another letter.

Dear Ingo,

Once again, I realized nobody can live my life for me. Nobody can help me, but sometimes I still have hope for the perfect solution. To find *the* cure for waiting, suffering, and all the other bullshit.

Today I know there is no such thing. Even the psychologist I saw doesn't know how to help me. I study psychology, and then psychology can't help me in my darkest hours. How sad. Maybe I should do something else after my transplant? Something nice. Something that has nothing to do with diseases, misery, or

> problems of other people. Maybe.
>
> Ugh, I don't know. I feel so lost. I'm not waiting anymore like a crazy person. I don't imagine my life after transplant anymore; I just exist in a vacuum. Figuratively and literally spoken.
>
> Did you also feel like that sometimes? Despite your wish list? The feeling of not being able to grab on to anything anymore? That everything is just falling apart around you and leaving nothing but vast emptiness behind?
>
> I could really use a little cheer-up. A push upward, a highlight, some light. These things exist in life, don't they? — Your slowly-dissolving-and-becoming-part-of-her-surrounding niece

The little cheer-up came. Though not in the shape of a cure for endless waiting, but in the shape of another checkup appointment in Hannover. Anamnesis and recommendations my doctor jotted down read like the following:

Overall, a clear improvement after the hospital and rehabilitation measures. Physiotherapy and exercising are possible again; liver is only partly functioning; blood sugar levels have improved, but the patient is still underweight. The arterial blood gas test shows respiratory failure (respiratory failure develops when the lung muscles aren't strong enough to supply the lungs with enough oxygen).

The next IV therapy should be done at a hospital; though the patient would prefer doing it at the rehab center in Amrum (Amrum is a German island in the North Sea). *We would support that wish. Right now, the next available time for a stay must be found. If treatment in Amrum isn't possible due to room availability, the patient should stay at our hospital.*

I was happy with what my doctors had to say. It sounded as if I was in good standing again. My weight was stable, my lung function sufficient to keep me alive, my next rehab on the horizon. Finally, I had something to look forward to again. A reason to keep going, other than staying alive: another rehab. I was excited until my doctors put things straight:

"We still would like you to consider being listed as high urgency," said one of them with a serious face. "You might seem stable now, but it's an illusion. You are suffering from respiratory failure, and your liver is barely doing what it's supposed to do. If you catch another stomach virus, or even a simple cold, you won't make it to your transplant."

Again, it was my sister who was with me at the hospital and heard my doctors raise the question of a high-urgency listing. Again.

I looked at her. She looked at me. We both knew what I would decide to do, but I wasn't ready this time to decide by myself. I wanted to talk this through with my parents. High urgency, yes or no. Should I wait the rest of my time in the hospital and hopefully get organs quicker? Or should I keep waiting at home, risking a longer wait time I might not survive?

"Do I have to decide right now?" I asked.

Both of my doctors shook their heads.

"No," said the one who had raised the topic, "it can wait, but not too long. Time is running out. It would be better for us to be proactive than wait until it's too late."

I looked at my two doctors and for the first time thought about how shitty the situation must feel for them. Doctors were supposed to save lives, and we were apparently running out of time.

If they felt emotional or defeated in that moment, they didn't show it. Emotions were reserved for being at home, not the hospital. It applied not only to patients but to doctors as well.

After our visit, we sat downstairs again in the shopping street, in front of the café, my sister eating a cheese sandwich, and me a Hawaii toast without pineapple. As always.

"They definitely know how to throw a party," my sister said while brushing crumbs off her shirt and pants. "After everything you have done, we are back at high urgency listing."

"Hm." I shoved the last bite of Hawaii toast without Hawaii into my mouth.

"If they could at least tell you how long you'd have to wait on high urgency, how many months or weeks you'd have to live in the hospital," my sister continued, putting her curly blond hair back into a ponytail, "then I'd say it's worth it."

I nodded. "Yeah, but they can't. And I don't want to live the rest of my life in a hospital room. If I don't survive the transplant, I have spent my last days, weeks, months even, inside a hospital. That just can't happen."

"You prefer to risk dying than staying in a hospital?" My sister raised one of her brows at me. She looked just like our mom when she did that.

"Have you ever eaten lunch in a hospital?" I asked in return. "I'd risk *your* life for not having to ever eat it again."

My sister smiled, though it was short-lived.

"No high urgency then? Are you sure?" she asked.

"In case I die . . ." I stood up, brushing crumbs off my own clothes the same way my sister had done, "I don't want to look back onto three months of wasted time in the hospital. If I die, I want to die happy. And happy only exists outside of these walls."

With that, my sister could only agree.

She dropped me off at my parents' on our way back home and, after a short explanation, they, too, agreed with my decision. No high urgency listing. Either I would survive my normal wait time, or not.

While my mom cleaned the kitchen, I sat in Dad's office and wrote another letter. It seemed so easy for me to decide against the high urgency listing, but it wasn't. I knew I took a huge risk in saying no. I was risking my life to have more fun during my wait time, but I didn't know what else to base my decision on. No matter what I decided, I didn't get a guarantee it would be the right one. Everything, no matter what I did, was in God's hands. God's hands, fate's hands, whoever was responsible. I never considered myself a very religious person. I believed, but I wasn't sure *what* I believed in. Maybe there was a God up there in heaven looking down on me, and all I had to do was trust. But could I?

Dear Ingo,

I will shock you today. I'm sorry, but can you tell me if God exists? Some higher power, some higher justice? A higher reason for it all? An old man with a long, white beard, sitting on a throne in the clouds, feet up, deciding before dinner how long my wait time should be? And if I'll survive?

You know, I don't believe in God, but I believe in something. I believe there is a higher reason for it all. I believe I don't just live without direction, without, let's say, being loved by God. But at the same time, I ask myself: *Why does he let me suffer for so long? Why do I have to decide for or against a high urgency listing?* What would God say if I could ask him: *Why am I still waiting to begin with? Why me? What did I do to deserve this?*

I don't want to start a quarrel with God, that feels awfully like bad karma, but on the other hand, I can't help myself. I want to scream at him, shout, curse, cuss, and show him how bad I feel and how much I deserve to be the next in line. High urgency or not. Or at least get an answer from him to the question of "Why?" If I could just understand.

I don't know where to leave all my frustration, doubt, and fear. Who to talk to when I feel so left alone with decisions no one should ever have to make—ever. — Your struggling-more-with-life-than-with-death niece

In German, we have a saying—*Reif für die Insel*—which means "ready for the island." No, it doesn't mean you're oiled up with sunscreen and ready for a beach vacation. It means, "I'm *oh-so ready* for the island and can't wait to get some time off from everything." On August 28, my mom and I were *reif für die Insel*. We packed our things and left for Amrum, where my second rehab would take place. Finally.

It was only luck that my wish had come true, that I could go to Amrum. Another patient hadn't been able to start her rehab as planned and as a result I had gotten her place, room, and bed. For once I had been granted all the luck in the world. It felt like I had won a beach vacation in an all-inclusive hotel, together with my mom. This time, she would stay the whole two weeks I would spend in rehab. It would be amazing. I couldn't wait.

To get to the island of Amrum, we had to take the ferry. Since it was past the summer holidays and past the main tourist season, the lines at the ferry dock weren't long. We waited about thirty minutes before the next ferry docked, ready to take the next line of cars over to Amrum. During season, one could easily wait two hours for a ferry ride.

Our short wait time for the ferry I spent in the car, eyes closed, breathing in the salty ocean air blowing in through the open window, dozing and trying to sustain as much energy for the ferry ride itself as possible. I already felt exhausted from doing nothing other than sitting beside my mom in the car, watching her drive, and climbing stairs on every stop we made.

We stopped a few times beside the Autobahn because we either needed more snacks or I needed to use the restroom. And every time the restrooms were either down the stairs or up the stairs. Which meant, either on my way back from or on my way to the restroom, I had to climb them.

On our last stop, facing the last set of stairs, I was ready to either pee my pants or just sit down and cry. I didn't want to climb stairs anymore that left me breathless, made me cough my lungs out, and invited unwelcome stares from everyone around me. Why couldn't one of these damn restrooms be on ground level? Why not?

I didn't pee my pants. I also made it up the last set of stairs, but I truly was close to tears. Sheer exhaustion can do that to you.

Once on the ferry I realized *those* restrooms were also downstairs. Down very narrow and steep stairs, but the ninety minutes of our ferry ride passed tearless. Most of that time I spent outside on the deck, watching the waves crash against the bow of the ship, the seagulls flying above, and the shore of Amrum growing bigger and bigger the closer we got.

Halfway, my mom brought two cups of steaming hot coffee outside, which she had gotten from the inside cafeteria, until we had to wrap up and get back to our car, because we were about to set foot onto Amrum. Finally.

I loved Amrum at first sight. Wherever I looked, I saw thatched cottages in front of white sand dunes. Beachgrass covered the dunes; they swayed in the wind, gulls swaying with them a few yards above. The lighthouse of Amrum rose into the sky in front of Amrum's main city, Nebel, or "fog" in English. When my eyes weren't locked on the sand dunes or cottages, I saw purplish heath that seemed to cover all the rest of the island.

Amrum is a rather small island, only about six miles long and a mile and a half wide, which meant the rehab center wasn't far. We passed the lighthouse, we arrived in Nebel, and a few minutes later, we were there. At the rehab center called Satteldüne, or "saddle dune" in English.

The Satteldüne looked from the outside a little bit like a tuberculosis sanatorium from the 1920s. Multiple, square, red brick buildings fused together, standing in a long line, representing medical care and professionalism. After all, this rehab center was specialized for patients with cystic fibrosis. It was supposed to look professional, but I still felt a little bit intimidated by it. What if they wouldn't let me decide what kind of therapies I wanted to do, but would tell me what I had to do? What if the rehab here would be completely different from the one I had experienced in St. Peter-Ording and I wouldn't like it? What if, what if, what if.

"Do you think these are rooms for patients?" my mom asked, interrupting my line of worries. She pointed up at the endless line of huge windows that followed us on our way to the entrance.

"If they are," I said, grateful for the distraction, "I hope I get one of those. You might even be able to see the sea from those rooms."

"Pretty nice." My mom nodded in agreement and held the door open for me to enter.

I did not get one of those rooms looking out to the sea, as most of them were offices. The rooms for the patients were by far not as fancy-looking. They, too, radiated the flair of a sanatorium from the 1920s, but I still felt at home pretty quickly, because I was surrounded by patients with the same disease and roughly the same age. In St. Peter-Ording, all the patients had been much older than me. Twenty-three-year-olds normally didn't go to rehab. But since all the patients in Amrum had CF, and medical problems from birth on, the overall age was way lower. All of us knew our way around a hospital, were coughing all the time, too skinny, doing IV therapy; some were even waiting for an organ transplant, same as me. But never mind how many life stories I heard—none of the other patients was waiting for a lung *and* liver transplant. Everyone on the waiting list *only* needed new lungs, and all of them were in better shape than me.

It was tough realizing after a few meals together with my new friends that I truly had drawn the shitty end of the stick. I knew it, and everyone else knew it too. Whenever we sat down and ate together, I could feel their doubt regarding my chance of survival. I was not isolated or treated like an outcast, not at all, but I could feel the distance between myself and them. As if everyone scooched aside so as not to be too close to the dying one.

What I had never seen in the eyes of my parents, I couldn't make unseen in the eyes of the other patients. I was way too skinny. I was weak, constantly exhausted, and barely holding on to the life that was left. For the first time, I wasn't sure anymore if my stubbornness, and my refusal to die, would be enough. I always knew I was close to death—latest after the stomach virus I had barely survived—but I never thought I would find myself in the situation where I wasn't able to do anything about it, other than accept death's proximity with a simple shrug.

As a result, I refused all group therapies. I didn't want to do yoga, breathing therapy, or movement together with the other, healthier patients. I only did private therapy sessions, and my doctors let me. No one tried to convince me to spend more time with others, to be more involved, or act more social. I was allowed to spend my remaining time the way I wanted to. Alone. With my mom. In private therapy. My doctors had little hope I would make it past my transplant and wanted me to enjoy my time in Amrum as much as I could. And I did, mostly because my doctors in Amrum had a completely different view of how IV antibiotics should be administered.

In Amrum, they simply injected the antibiotics into the vein. Like having blood drawn, just the other way around. No blood was sucked out of my vein, but antibiotics were inserted into it. Never had I seen anything like it.

In every hospital I had ever spent a night in, the nurses had warned me not to let the antibiotic IV drip too fast into my vein, but in Amrum, they injected it. It took two minutes to inject my IVs, compared to an hour and a half when administered by a slow drip.

Because of this, I had a lot of free time that I spent with my mom. Every afternoon, after my injected IV, my mom and I took small walks along the shore. Often with our shoes off, feet touching the cold waves coming in, collecting shells, and sometimes resting in one of the hooded beach chairs that were sprinkled along the shoreline.

A hooded beach chair is called *strandkorb*, or beach basket in German, and one of the most iconic items one can find along the shore of the North Sea. Every sea resort plasters the shore with these hooded, windbreaking chairs, constructed from wicker, wood panels, and canvas, and everyone loves to sit in or take pictures of them. Same as me.

I often sat in a *strandkorb* when I was too tired to walk, with my feet lying on the pullout footrest. I loved watching my mom stroll along the beach. It was good for both of us to have a little time by ourselves. Letting worries take form and then allowing the wind from the sea to blow them away across the mainland. It truly did feel like some sort of beach vacation. Like one last beach vacation, which made me cherish it even more.

On my last night in Amrum, the clinic had a special event planned. Former patients were invited from all over Germany to join the clinic and its patients for a barbecue in the sand dunes.

Many came. Many people with CF who seemed so healthy and normal that evening. They arrived at the barbecue, chatted with other patients, laughed with doctors, ate, and drank without having a single coughing fit.

While the moon shined from above, every twenty seconds the lighthouse scurried its cone of light over the dunes; to us, it felt magical. A perfect last day, even though I couldn't help but envy every guest who had come. I looked at them, imagined them having a normal life where they went to work every day, drove around in their cars to faraway barbecues, and now ate bratwurst and drank beer without a worry in the world.

I wanted to be one of those former patients. I wanted to arrive at a rehab clinic and not come for needles, IVs, and therapy, but only to eat a brat and then drive back home. What a privilege to be one of those. It felt so alien to me, I couldn't even imagine.

My rehab ended, and this time, I was at peace with it. I had enjoyed my time on the island very much, but I was also glad to be back home. I was ready to sit back down on my parents' sofa in front of the TV and let time simply pass by.

Suddenly I didn't feel the need to fill the life I still had with anything anymore. I was content with where I was. Still alive. Still breathing. Still hoping for a miracle that would never come. The call, the call that fitting organs were there for me . . . we weren't waiting for it anymore. We had waited for so long, we had nursed hope for so long without success, without ever saying it out loud, that all of us had made peace with the fact that all the things I had wished for would never come.

That's why on October 20, Martina jumped into her car and drove three hours to come see me. For one last time. To say her goodbyes.

I don't remember anything from that visit. Not one word, not one tear, absolutely nothing. As if I was still there but already on my way, leaving this world behind. Or literally too tired to give a shit.

When Martina left that evening to drive back home, she stopped somewhere on her way, on the side of the road, and cried. She was sure she had seen me for the last time. When she got home, she wrote in her diary: "Inka, please stay!"

14

EXISTING

The following weeks passed by in a steady but otherwise vacuum-filled manner. We reduced my physiotherapy to twice a week, as I couldn't handle more than that. I was in a constant state of exhaustion, every day ready to go back to bed right after breakfast. I didn't do much other than watching TV, eating, and sleeping. I didn't communicate with my friends, only a few phone calls here and there I couldn't avoid. I didn't write anything in my diary. I didn't pay attention to anything around me. I was just there. Surviving one day after another. Not waiting for organs anymore. Just being, and nothing else.

On November 13, I had another checkup appointment in Hannover. This time, my mom had to put me in a wheelchair to get me from one doctor to another. Walking the long halls of the hospital was not possible anymore.

After the visit, I started another IV therapy—this one from home. Other than that, nothing changed. I still didn't want to be listed as high urgency, which meant my doctors were not able to help me any further. From now on, it was a sole race against time. Would I be able to survive until organs were available, or would I not make it in time?

On my first evening of my IV therapy, I sat down once again in my dad's office and wrote another letter to Ingo. I had to leave my emotions somewhere, and I didn't dare leave them with my parents or friends. I just couldn't tell my parents how I didn't care anymore if I got transplanted or not. How I only wanted this endless suffering to end. Happily or not. Same as I couldn't tell my friends how all the things they wanted to do with me together after my transplant were nothing more than soap bubbles on a windy day. There were no dreams anymore. Just an endless line of endless days, an endless line of slowly dripping IVs. (God, I missed Amrum and their shoot-it-straight-up-the-vein approach.)

> Dear Ingo,
>
> I started another IV therapy. Every time I start another one, I ask myself: *Will this be the last IV therapy I ever have to do in my life?* And then the next one is scheduled.
>
> But you know what, it doesn't really matter anymore. Nothing matters anymore. I wrap myself in indifference, and I have to say, it feels good not giving a shit about anything. Like a protective bubble. I don't wait anymore, I don't despair anymore, I only exist.
>
> I know, I sound awfully depressed, but you don't have to worry. I'm just feeling empty. Too tired to feel anything anymore. That's why I simply exist. One day after another. It's like sleeping, sleeping until it goes on. Is the place beside you on cloud nine still free? Not that I don't have anywhere to sit in heaven.

> A few days ago, I talked with my mom about my funeral. I don't know how we got to that topic, but we talked about it. I want everyone to wear normal clothes to my funeral, nothing black. It should be colorful. And if it rains, no black umbrellas like in a TV drama. When I look down from heaven, I want to see colorful umbrellas instead of black octagons.
>
> That reminds me, I don't even know what your funeral looked like. I only know you were cremated because you wanted the cancer to die with you. I understand that. But I think I don't want to be cremated. I want to become part of earth again, the traditional worm way. Become part of the circle again. Weird, right? I never thought I'd care what would happen after I'm dead. Dead is dead. But now it feels like death has become a part of my life. Like something that needs planning. I want to be buried in the family grave. I don't want to lay somewhere alone and rot away. I want to rest in peace where you were lying down. To walk the last steps with you together. Even in death, I don't want to be alone. — Your not-always-sure-about-her-own-feelings niece

My IV was done, and more days passed by—uneventful as usual. Then Christmas was on the horizon.

And this time, I had no chance of escaping it.

We celebrated, as we did every year except 2001, as a family at my parents' house. My sister's friend joined us, as she didn't have anywhere else to go that year, and to my surprise, I truly enjoyed it. My dad oversaw cooking and music selection. I decorated the tree early in the afternoon. My mom and Tina set the table and the presents under the tree.

From the outside, it looked like a normal Christmas. On the inside, everyone knew this would be my last Christmas if I didn't get transplanted soon. Because of it, everyone was quieter than usual. No loud outbursts of laughter, no fighting over the volume of the stereo system, and only a small amount of wine and champagne. Most of our emotions seemed to stay on the inside that holiday. The outside a façade of calm and normal.

As a present for my mom, I got a silver angel from Martina. Martina made brooches of angels that one could either wear on a jacket or hang in a picture frame on the wall. I knew it would look perfect in their living room, and an angel fit perfectly to my mom. She had been my guardian angel for all this time. I would never be able to thank her enough, but an angel was at least a start.

My mom was sure I didn't give her a thank-you but a parting gift. That I was preparing everyone for my final goodbye.

I wished I would have known her thoughts when she unwrapped my gift and had tears rolling down her cheeks. Then I could have told her how the topic of goodbye hadn't even crossed my mind yet. I knew I was dying, but at the same time, I repeatedly only concentrated on surviving the next day. And surviving the next day had always seemed possible so far.

The holidays rolled by as any of the other days before did. The only difference was that there was no physiotherapy during the holidays (physio was closed), which is why I walked around the neighborhood with my mom instead. My dad spent more time in the kitchen than usual to cook up a few special dishes for the holidays, to keep my appetite up 24/7. Other than that, nothing but boredom—same old, same old—until the evening of December 27.

Like every Friday evening, my mom and I sat in front of the TV and watched one of the Friday evening talk shows we loved so much. This evening, one of the guests was a heart transplant surgeon from Hannover. From *my* Hannover. The same hospital I was listed at for my transplant.

"Too bad it's not a lung transplant surgeon," I said while settling in on the sofa, a pile of snacks by my side.

"True." My mom agreed and turned up the volume a notch. "I still want to hear it though," she said, and I got the hint. I placed my oxygen back under my nose and waved my dad good night when he passed the living room on his way to bed. I was quiet, even though it wasn't the doctor's turn yet. A German alpine skier who had won a medal in the Winter Olympics earlier that year was talking about her medal and growing up in the mountains.

I didn't really care. I paid more attention to my snack bowl when my cell, lying in my dad's office, suddenly rang.

My mom looked at me, forehead wrinkled.

"Who is calling you now?" she asked as if I should know. "It's past ten. Don't they know this is your transplant cell? No one should call that late other than the hospital."

I just shrugged, pulled the oxygen off my face, and got up to take the call. Whoever it was, at least I didn't have to listen to alpine skiing tales anymore.

In my dad's office, I pulled his chair out, sat down, and grabbed my cell phone, but I didn't recognize the number.

"Rasch," I said, as it's common in Germany to answer the phone with only stating your last name. (My maiden name was Rasch.)

"Good evening, Ms. Rasch," a man on the other end greeted me. "This is Dr. K from Hannover calling. How are you feeling today?"

My heart skipped a beat, and a huge smile appeared on my face. This was Hannover. Calling after 10:00 p.m. to ask me how I felt. This could only mean one thing.

"I feel good," I said, way calmer than I felt.

"No fever. No cold. Stomach flu, anything?"

"Nope," I said. "All good."

I heard a "Hmm" coming through the phone and could almost see the doctor on the other end nodding to himself.

"We have an offer for organs for you." He finally said what I already knew. "Do you still want to be transplanted?"

"What?" I laughed. I had not expected that question. "Of course," I said. "That's what I've been waiting for since the last fifteen months."

I pressed the phone into my ear, not to miss anything else the doctor had to say, and turned around to see if by miracle my mom was standing in the doorframe hearing what I was hearing because I almost couldn't believe it. Organs. For me. After all I had been through. After believing I would never get a second chance in life—everything had changed from one second to another. From death to hope. From nothing to everything. I wasn't sure if I felt too hot or was freezing, but I could feel a smile spreading all over my face and lighting up the night. Bringing the Christmas spirit back to our home.

"Yes," I said once again, just to be sure to be heard, "I still want to get transplanted." I wondered if there were patients out there who weren't sure when the time came. Who'd say, "No, I'd rather die. Thank you very much though. Have a nice night"?

"Great," the doctor said. "Please stay close to your phone. Soon someone from the transplant office is going to call you to arrange your transport to Hannover. Don't take any measures into your own hands. We will take care of everything. Any more questions?"

I couldn't think of anything besides *I got organs, I got organs, I got organs,* but then one question still came to mind.

"Do you think they will fly me to Hannover or drive me in an ambulance? I've never flown before. I would love to fly to Hannover."

Now it was the doctor's turn to laugh.

"Honestly, I don't know." He chuckled. "That's all arranged by the ladies of the transplant office. We have no say in that."

Fair enough. We said goodbye, and I went back to the living room, the stupid smile still plastered on my face, my mom still fuming on the sofa.

"Who was it?" she asked. "Who had the audacity to call this late on your transplant phone?"

"Hannover," I said.

Her forehead wrinkled in disbelief. "Hannover? But I heard you laughing."

"Yes," I said. "Because it's happening."

15

FINALLY

The next few hours passed in a blur. First, my mom went upstairs to wake up my dad. None of us cared anymore to hear what the heart transplant surgeon from Hannover had to say. The TV blared on, but its audience was gone.

While my mom woke up my dad, I called my sister. She was still awake and immediately jumped into her car and drove to Hannover to meet us there.

After that was taken care of, I went to brush my teeth as thoroughly as possible. With floss and everything. No idea why my dental hygiene was that important to me at that moment, but I thought: *Who knows when I'll be able to brush my teeth again, might as well.*

And then all three of us sat in front of the TV again, waiting for the call to tell us what would happen next. My dad took one last picture of me, as I was sitting with a huge smile on the sofa, and then finally my phone rang.

"We will be picked up by an ambulance," I told my parents after I hung up, "and the ambulance—drumroll, please—will drive us to the airport in Düsseldorf from where we will *flyyyy* to Hannover."

I did a pathetic dance move, some jazz hands, and grinned at my mom. She was terrified of flying. This would be fun.

"Great," was all she had to say.

My dad said nothing, but his grin said everything.

The wait time for the ambulance was short. Thirty minutes after my phone call had ended, the ambulance arrived, ready to drive me and my mom to the airport. My dad, as always, stayed home. Frist of all, there wouldn't be enough room for all of us in the Learjet that would fly me to Hannover, and second, as I had mentioned before, my dad and hospitals just didn't match. He knew it, we knew it, and all of us had made peace with it, but that also left me with having to say goodbye to him right then.

We stood behind the ambulance parked on our deserted street, only lit by a streetlamp, and I was about to climb inside and get comfortable on the gurney when my dad opened his arms and embraced me in a crushing hug.

"I love you," he mumbled into my hair.

"Me too," I answered, and that was it. He released me, I climbed into the ambulance, and my mom sat in the co-pilot's seat. The EMT closed the door, and we were on our way.

I was grateful that our goodbye had been short. There was no need to say a million words, only three: I love you.

Peering out the small back window of the ambulance, I watched my dad and my parents' house grow smaller and smaller, and couldn't help but ask myself:

Will I ever see all of this again? Will I ever see my dad again, or had this short moment outside in their driveway with him been our last? Our last hug? Our last spoken words to each other?

I clenched my teeth, shook my head, and stopped any thoughts altogether. I wouldn't think of what could be. I wouldn't think ahead,

I wouldn't get emotional, teary, none of that. I was on my way to get transplanted. Nothing else mattered. If I'd make it, or if I didn't, wasn't important right now. All that mattered was my transplant. That's where my focus was. Only there and nowhere else.

"Everything okay?" the EMT asked. "Do you need oxygen or want to lie down?"

"All okay," I said. "And no, I don't need anything. Sitting is fine."

The EMT went back to filling out papers, and I went back to looking out the back window.

One. Step. At. A. Time.

We entered the airport through its back entrance. A huge metal gate was opened in front of us, and the ambulance driver waved a thank-you to the security guard while we drove past parked private jets directly up to our Learjet. Its doors were already open, a short staircase extended, the pilot, his co-pilot, and two EMTs waiting for me.

"Do you want to stay on the gurney?" my EMT asked, "or do you want to walk up to the jet yourself?"

"Myself," I said with full conviction. *This might be my one and only flight.* I wanted to enjoy it. I wanted to pretend I was a famous person, flying to my next book signing. I did not want to lie on a gurney like some kind of sick person.

My EMT helped me to get off the gurney, I stepped out of the ambulance, and together with my mom we climbed the stairs to greet one of the jet's EMTs, ready to welcome us onboard.

"Good evening," he said. Shaking my hand and then Mom's hand. "We didn't expect you to still be that mobile after we heard we will be flying a patient to their lungs and liver transplant. Seems like this will be a relaxing flight. Welcome onboard."

"Hi," was all I could muster after climbing the four steep jet stairs. I was already out of breath.

The EMT showed me where to sit at the back of the plane. Past the now empty gurney on my right was a small cushioned bench, in front of it a table, where my mom and I sat down. It did feel like flying in a private jet. Truly like being a celebrity of some sorts. Only the champagne was missing.

"Do you need oxygen?" the EMT asked me.

"No," I said. "I want to fly without." I didn't want to taint this flight by having tubes stuck under my nose. No way.

"If you change your mind," he said, "let me know." And then to my mom: "Would you like a cup of coffee? We also still have some cookies I can offer."

Coffee? I was impressed and a little bit jealous. I wasn't allowed to drink or eat anything in preparation for the anesthesia I'd be getting soon, but of course, my mom couldn't say no.

"I'll take a cup of coffee and cookies." She grinned in my direction. "Flying might not be that bad after all."

The flight was short. About ninety minutes. The whole time I was glued to the window, looking down onto sleeping and lit up Germany, thinking of nothing. I didn't think of what was ahead. I didn't think of my dad at home, my sister on her way, or my mom slurping coffee next to me while chatting with the EMTs. I just looked down. Watched cities pass by and tried to enjoy every minute of this unique experience. Who knew if I would ever fly again. Who knew if I would survive the next twenty-four hours.

"Prepare for landing," the pilot announced over the intercom, and everything snapped back to what it was. Me on my way to my transplant. Being terminally ill and not some celebrity on her way to a book signing. Coffee mugs were stored, cookies wrapped up, and just like that, we were all back to reality.

When we arrived at the medical school of Hannover, my sister was already there, waiting for us, reading trashy celebrity magazines and drinking, of course, coffee.

"Finally." She sighed when she saw us coming toward her. "Never thought my Mercedes would be that much faster than a Learjet, but okay."

We all hugged and looked at each other, unsure of what to say or if there even was anything to say; luckily, there wasn't much time for any of that. My sister wasn't the only one waiting. The nurses and doctors who were assigned to prep me bustled about.

"Okay," one of the nurses said to let us all know I had more important things to do than hug and be speechless. "We need to get going and get you prepped. First, we need an X-ray of your lungs and abdomen. We have to draw blood, shave you down, and you need to sign a few papers before the show starts. Ready?"

I nodded, a bit overwhelmed by what was happening, but since the ball was rolling, there was nothing to do anymore than run after it.

My nurse placed me in a wheelchair, and we were on our way to check off all the items on her prep list. My mom and sister would wait for me.

"She'll be back in about an hour," my nurse told them, and we took off around the next corner.

The prep was quick. X-rays—done. Blood drawn—almost a gallon of it. Never had anyone taken that much blood from me in one sitting before. And then the shaving. Every tiny hair on my abdomen and chest had to be gone. I felt like cattle being prepped for slaughter. Everything was done in a very detached manner. There were no comforting words, no pitiful looks, only appointments that had to be completed as efficiently and quickly as possible. The only good thing about it was that I didn't have any time for emotions either. I was on the road to my transplant, and no one would step on the brakes for me to freak out about it.

When I was done with everything, I was placed in a hospital bed and parked in the sitting area of the post-transplant floor where my mom and sister were already waiting for me. They had gotten as comfortable as possible on a sofa, illuminated by the lights of a fake, blue, and awful-looking Christmas tree. Both looked exhausted.

"Can I bring you anything?" the nurse asked me. "A sleeping pill or some Dormicum?"

I looked at my mom, momentarily confused, but it was my sister who answered my unasked question.

"She means an I-don't-give-a-shit pill. Dormicum will make you sleepy and not worry anymore. You know, the kind of medication patients get before surgery to calm them down?"

"Oh." I nodded. I did know Dormicum and did know I did not want it.

"I'm fine," I said. "I won't need anything."

"Let one of the nurses on the floor know if you change your mind," my nurse said and left us alone.

"I'd like an I-don't-give-a-shit pill," my mom said before we all settled back and tried to sleep a little. I had been told it would take a while before my actual transplant would start. We had to wait.

As always.

Around 6:00 a.m., things started to move again. First, the surgeon who would later transplant my lungs came by to introduce himself and talk us through the steps of a bilateral lung transplant. Just so all of us knew what to expect. Honestly, I didn't care how they would exchange my lungs, but my mom and sister were all ears.

"We will pick you up at nine," he said once he was done with his explanations. "Oh, and I saw the pair of lungs you'll get. They look great."

He waved a quick goodbye and went on his way to get ready for my transplant.

"Great-looking lungs," I said and held up my thumb.

"At least you will get *something* great-looking," my sister added, and we both laughed.

My mom raised her eyebrows.

"He means the condition of the lungs," she said. "They are healthy lungs, great lungs."

"Great and great-looking," my sister and I said at the same time and exchanged a high five. We were all ready. We were all eager to get going and not wait any longer. Eager and scared.

Shortly after, the liver transplant surgeon stopped by as well.

"Wow," he said when he interrupted another giggle my sister and I shared. "Good spirits this morning. I like it."

He, too, introduced himself, explained the steps of a liver transplant, and the extent of the scars I'd carry from it.

"It'll look like a huge Mercedes star on your belly," he explained and demonstrated the dimensions of it on his belly.

We all nodded. None of us had ever asked about the scars such a procedure would leave behind. Scars had never come to my mind. Dying, yes. Scars, not at all.

"We will pick you up around nine," he said, confirming what the lung transplant surgeon had said before. We were left alone once again.

"I don't want to hear a single word about Mercedes stars from the two of you," my mom said, raising her index finger at us.

"Still," I said, exchanging a look with my sister, "a Jaguar would have been way cooler."

"As long as it's not a Kia," my sister added, and we burst out laughing again.

It felt so good to be silly, to joke around. Not thinking of the magnitude of this moment. The chances were high I wouldn't survive the transplant. This could easily be my last moments with my mom and sister, and there was no better way than spending them laughing, joking, ignoring reality, and annoying our mom. It helped me to stay clear, focused, and alert till the last moment. No I-don't-give-a-shit pill was needed. Not for me. I wasn't scared. I was ready.

At 9:00 a.m. sharp, I was picked up and rolled, still in my bed, through half of the hospital. We even drove along the shopping street. It was still empty at that time, but the café was already open. I wondered . . .

If I'd ever eat another Hawaii toast without Hawaii here . . .

If I'd ever sit here again with a café au lait in hand, talking to my mom . . .

If I'd ever...

We turned the corner, and I, once again, banned all thoughts directed to the future. It didn't matter what would be. Only now mattered. Only my transplant mattered.

When we arrived at the prep room, all jokes were gone. The moment had come when I had to say goodbye to my mom and my sister.

"I don't . . ." My mom started, but I cut her off immediately.

"Let's just hug and you leave," I said, reaching out my arms. I wanted no thinking ahead. No asking myself if I would ever see my mom again. None of that. Just a hug, a wave, and a closed door to keep all our emotions at bay.

"Okay, bye," I said after our long hug and shooed her out of the room. One done. One more to go, but my sister stayed a little longer. We didn't say anything. We both watched all the movements around me. How someone placed the EKG electrodes on my chest. Another person placed a blood pressure cuff around my arm, while another person turned up the oxygen flow under my nose and taped the electrode for the oximeter around my ring finger. And then it was also time for my sister to say goodbye.

"See you later," she said, pressed my shoulder, and left.

"What?" I said, trying to get her back, but then I just smiled instead. No drama indeed. *See you later.* It sounded as if I only had to survive a wart removal. Gotta love my sister.

Outside the prep room, my sister collapsed into my mom's arms and they cried together. All coolness, all composure gone. The fear, that this might have been the last time they had seen me alive, was very real to them. Thank God it wasn't to me. I was busy helping the nurses around me getting this transplant on its way. Grateful to keep my mind occupied.

"We will lift you over to the operation table now," one of the nurses told me, then grabbed my bedsheet, but I stopped him.

"I can climb over myself," I said, already sitting up to get over there.

"You didn't get a sedative before they brought you here?" he asked in surprise.

"You mean an I-don't-give-a-shit pill?"

Everyone laughed inside the prep room.

"No," I said. "This is my transplant. This is important. I can't just pass out and let you guys do everything."

More laughing, and a relaxed breeze went through the room while I climbed onto the hard operation table. I got a surgical hat placed over my hair, someone introduced themselves, someone stroked my covered head, the blood pressure cuff tightened around my upper arm, and I could hear my heartbeat broadcasted throughout the room.

I concentrated on my breathing, tried to force myself to calm down, to lower the speed of my heartbeat, when another person in a green gown took a seat beside my head and introduced himself as the anesthesiologist.

"I'm here to place a venous access into your arm, and then we'll administer the anesthesia."

"Okay." There was nothing else to say, so I watched him search for a vein he could use. It didn't take him long to decide on one.

"We will take this one," he told me. "But before I place the venous access, I will locally numb the spot so it won't be that painful when I poke you."

"You'll locally numb the area around my vein?" I had to repeat what he said.

"Yes . . ." Now he was the confused one. "Why wouldn't I?"

"I have gotten millions of venous accesses placed over the years. Many as a kid and never, ever has anyone numbed the spot beforehand."

It looked like he smiled at me behind his surgical mask.

"And *I* never, ever had anyone complain about it before their transplant."

Now it was my turn to smile.

Later, after my transplant was done, my mom and sister heard all about how much fun everyone had with me during the preparation. How it didn't happen often that patients still made jokes about local anesthesia before their transplant.

When the venous access was placed, the anesthesiologist grabbed a syringe with a milky-looking liquid inside.

"This is the anesthesia," he told me. "I will administer it now. It might burn a little, but it shouldn't last too long."

He plugged the syringe into my venous access and started to push the plunger down.

It burned like hell. Local sedation, my ass.

Someone asked me something, but I couldn't answer anymore. A deep humming noise filled my ears, and then everything went black.

16

Oblivion

It was 9:55 a.m. when the surgeon set the scalpel under my right breast and made the first cut. The transplant was underway.

Shortly after, my mom texted everyone:

> **December 28, 2002, 10:02 a.m.**
> Inka is in the operation room since 9 am. Please don't call. I will write again.

I didn't have any memories of my transplant surgery. I didn't see myself from above, lying on the table, hearing the surgeons talking; I didn't count the gauze they took back out from my open chest cavity and abdomen. What happened to me during the next eight hours can only be retold from the non-emotional operation report I received later.

The whole report read like an instruction manual for an organ transplant. Objectively, it described one step at the time, nothing more. It detailed when an artery was cut, if scar tissue had to be removed, if bleeding had to be stopped; how the new lungs actually looked, how much my old liver weighed, how much the new one weighed.

There were no tears once the complications arrived. When my circulatory system collapsed, my news lungs refused to deliver enough oxygen to my body. No one held their breath when the first clamps were removed, when I was disconnected from the heart-lung machine and then had to be stitched up in a state of emergency because suddenly my liver was failing. There was no emotion. Everyone just continued working.

Looking back, I felt the same lack of emotion as the report. I didn't feel much reading what a close call it was back then. I was under anesthesia. I didn't have to wait eight hours to hear back from a nurse that I had survived my transplant. I just slept while everyone else worried.

Due to all the stress, my sister threw up multiple times once she and my mom reached a hotel room they had booked.

Silke, inspired by the feeling of not being able to do anything, decided to drive, together with her boyfriend, to Hannover to be at least close to me. But she never made it to Hannover. Halfway, she called my mom to let her know she was on her way, but unfortunately, my sister picked up and made her turn back around *immediately*. No one in my family had the resources to also deal with the worry and presence of anybody else. Friends would be kept informed via texts but asked, unequivocally, to stay where they were and not come anywhere near Hannover Medical School. Silke included.

My roommate Aria called every friend of mine to inform them of what was happening, cried a few tears with most of them, but talking to each other helped pass the horrible hours of waiting to hear any news.

Martina turned to her diary instead. Holding on to the belief I would make it because I never gave up hope. Opposite to herself.

At 5:50 p.m., my liver transplant was complete. Intubated and stable, I was moved to ICU. A few hours later, my mom wrote her next text:

> **December 28, 2002, 7:59 p.m.**
> OP went well with small complications. Doctors are content. Inka is stable for now. We can go see her tomorrow around noon.

The next day, as announced by my mom, she and my sister were allowed to pay me a short visit in ICU. I didn't acknowledge either of them. I was still intubated, still had a tube running through my mouth and into my lungs, through which I was ventilated and therefore still sedated. Nobody likes to be fully awake when having a tube stuck down one's throat.

Their visit was short and unsatisfying. There I was, connected to a million tubes, not responding, looking like I was about to die but still somewhat alive. It seemed like there was more medical equipment than Inka in that bed. My sister counted fifteen infusions dripping different medications into my system.

It was heartbreaking to see. I was supposed to be fixed, ready to go with new organs onboard, but my body looked more than ever like it was about to give up.

And then I opened my eyes.

"She's awake," my mom said, scared and surprised at once, and then added: "Inka, it's us. Can you hear us?"

I could hear them, I could see them, but I wasn't aware of anything due to the sedation. I didn't know where I was, who I was, or anything else, but I did have something to say.

Because of the tube in my throat, I couldn't talk, but I showed them what I needed. I pointed at my leg and then acted as if I was falling asleep.

"Do you need a painkiller?" my sister asked, but no, that wasn't it.

Forcefully, I shook my head.

"Is it your leg?" My mom joined in, but again, that wasn't it.

A nurse came to help, but she had no idea what I was trying to say either, and I started to get angry. How stupid were they for not understanding what I was trying to say.

Again, I pointed at my leg, this time with more force, and then acted as if falling asleep. Three dumbfounded faces stared back at me.

It was probably a good thing I was still intubated and couldn't express my anger and therefore couldn't give my mom a flashback from the *last* time I had fought for my life by being nasty to everyone around me.

"How about," my sister said, "I spell the ABCs and you nod your head when I come to the right letter? That way you can spell out what you need."

I nodded, hesitantly, but okay, we could give it a try. I knew it would take some time, because what I wanted to spell was "syringe with sleeping medication" and the letter S was all the way at the end of the ABCs. It gets better: I had to spell it in German. In German, the sentence to spell was "*Spritze mit Schlafmittel.*" Same problem, same S, but whatever. If none of these idiots were able to understand my gestures, we would do it the slow way.

My sister started to recite the ABCs, and I spelled along. I was surprised I was able to spell. I didn't even know what was going on, but spelling I did know.

It felt like forever, but eventually everyone understood what I needed, the nurse injected me with some sleep medicine, and I waved a drowsy goodbye to my mom and sister. Finally, back to sleep. I was so grateful when everything slowly slipped away around me and I went back to oblivion. I didn't have to lie in my ICU bed, unable to move or get comfortable, unable to ask someone what was going on; I didn't have to experience complete helplessness while counting endless seconds, minutes, and hours filled with misery. I could just sleep and forget.

And sleep I did . . .

People are running past my bed and rushing out the glass door at the end of the hall onto the parking lot behind. It's after my transplant, I remember. Everything went well, I survived, but something is wrong. The atmosphere around me is too stressful, too charged for a hospital. Carefully, I look around. My bed is placed inside a nook in the hall. I'm not inside my room or in the ICU as I expected. I'm lying in the hallway! And then I hear gunshots, somewhere, farther away. Maybe two hallways down. The hospital is taken by force. The door at the end of the hallway, where just moments ago people escaped through, is now barricaded. Nobody will get in or out. One of the hostage-takers comes around the corner and slowly walks by my bed. A huge machine gun is hanging over his shoulder, but I try not to look at him, not to draw any attention to myself. Slowly I pull my legs closer, try to make myself smaller, try to vanish. Because I can't die like this, not here, not today. My parents will be crushed by despair knowing I survived my transplant but was shot by a stray bullet fired by one of the hostage-takers.

At the same time as I was trying to survive a hostage situation in my drug-induced dreams, the nurses around me fought for my life. I thrashed around in my bed. My blanket fell on the floor, my legs were all over the place, and then, to the horror of everyone around me, I pulled out the feeding tube that ran through my nose into my stomach. Pulled it all the way out in one swift motion.

"We need to tie her down," someone said. "We can't risk her pulling the breathing tube too."

"And increase her sedation," another one answered.

All my fighting was a reaction to my dreams, but no one suspected me of having nightmares. The sedatives I got were supposed to evoke happy dreams, sometimes even erotic ones, but apparently not for me. I was in survival mode, in and outside of my dreams.

The nurses around my bed are talking badly about me. Making fun of me behind my back. They even tie me up, "Just for fun," as they say and leave me, fixated onto the mattress under me. I try to scream and cuss at them, but they can't hear me. Eventually one of them comes back to my room and injects me with sleeping medication. Again, just for fun. I can't wait to tell my mom about all the awful things happening here. Once I wake up again. Once I'm awake.

On December 29, one day after my transplant, doctors performed another small operation on me. I had a small leak in my lungs, which was closed by a minor surgery.

I'm standing on a road, alone. It's evening, dark and rainy. I have no idea where I am or what I'm doing here. If I'm waiting for someone or got lost. A little stressed, I turn around, look up and down the deserted road, until I see a lit telephone booth. A man is standing inside of it. He's wearing a long, beige-brown coat and a hat with a brim. I can't see his face, but he looks like he's from the '70s. I watch him, how he hangs up the phone, opens the door of the telephone booth, and walks away in haste. Unsure, I watch him leave and suddenly know I must keep him in sight. I must follow him. Because only as long as I can see him, everything will be fine. As long as I can only see his back and not his face, nothing will happen to me.

Days later, when I was finally able to think clearly again, I told my mom about this dream and she was sure I had seen Ingo. Long coat, hat with a brim—that could have only been Ingo.

I had this dream multiple times during the first days after my transplant. It never occurred to me then that it was Ingo who visited me, but the dream itself always made me feel safe. Like I was on the right track.

> **December 29, 2002, 6:23 p.m.**
> Second OP (closing leak in the lungs) went without complications. Inka is stable. Doctors are content.

While I'm in ICU, the patient right next to me dies. He's an older guy, I don't know him, I don't really care, but then a team of surgeons arrives, cut him open, right there, right beside me, and harvest his organs. I'm horrified by what I see. Blood spills everywhere. Unneeded parts of his intestines fall on the ground, get trampled by the harvesting doctors, and no one seems to care. After they're done, the leftovers of the body are dumped onto the floor, like an empty shell pushed into a corner, where it just lays and rots. No one comes to clean it up. No one cares that this has been a human being once, that there are blood smears everywhere, nurses walking by every day, leaving bloody footprints behind. It's like a scene out of a Stephen King novel. And I'm one of the characters.

December 30, 2002, 9:03 a.m.
Night went without complications. I can visit her this midday. Assisted ventilation will continue for two more days.

Not all my dreams were filled with blood and gore. Many of them had, oddly enough, shower curtains in them. I dreamed how my sister helped another patient to shower while I was sitting alone in my bed, being jealous and feeling neglected. I dreamed of showering myself while being attacked by flip-flop frogs that clapped around and charged me with noisy vengeance. I had that dream multiple times. Frogs and shower curtains, what the hell.

Only once I was awake and had my glasses back on my nose again did I understand where those dreams had come from. Above my bed was a rail, which allowed curtains to be pulled between the beds in ICU. In ICU, you don't have your own room. The patients lay beside each other like sardines in a can. The only privacy there is comes from closing these curtains. From my perspective and with my limited vision, they had looked like shower curtains. Reality and weird dreams often went hand in hand.

> **December 30, 2002, 3:57 p.m.**
> Inka continues to be stable. Upcoming days will be crucial.

A nurse came to my bed to suck accumulated mucus out of my throat. Mucus simply accumulated when being on ventilation. This was done twice each day. I knew the procedure, I had it done multiple times before, but that day I was awake enough to know I didn't want it. It was not fun having someone stick a tube down your throat and let them suck the mucus out while you tried to keep your gag reflex under control. When she leaned over me, sucking tube in hand, I reached for it.

"Your hands stay down," she told me in a very stern voice. Stern enough that I didn't dare try again.

After I had pulled my feeding tube out of my mouth, every nurse was on edge when I lifted so much as a finger in the direction of my face. Nobody wanted to witness me pulling out my breathing tube too.

She exchanged one more stern look with me, letting me know this was not a joke, and put the sucking tube into my mouth, heading for my throat. When I bit down, I trapped the tube with my teeth so she couldn't move it forth a back.

"Haha, you bitch!" I wanted to shout. *"You won't shove that tube down my throat if I won't let you."*

I should have known that there was no self-determination in ICU.

I eventually did get the mucus sucked out of my throat. But my small victory remained.

> **December 31, 2002, 1:09 p.m.**
> Everything is stable. Liver works well. Assisted ventilation is still going.

When my mom drove back home that evening—home being the house of my aunt at that time—she found a cut-out article of that day's newspaper lying on the kitchen table. The title read: *A New Heart: A Gift for Life.* And the subtitle said: *In the middle of the night, one phone call ends the months-long wait. Lungs, heart, liver—an organ donor gives two terminally ill patients a second chance.*

My mom picked up the article, sat down, and started to read:

> *During the night of December 27 two patients will have their dream come true to get a second chance of life.*
>
> *10 pm: Eurotransplant calls the Hannover Medical School telling them: We have a heart, lungs and one liver for you.*
>
> *10:15 pm: Chief physician Dr. Martin Strüber., who isn't even working that day, mobilizes his transplant team. Then he goes back to bed, his cell right beside him.*

12:30 am: A team of surgeons from Hannover flies out to recover the organs. During a traffic accident multiple people were fatally injured. One of them was declared brain dead at a nearby hospital.

3:00 am: The team from Hannover determines that the organs of the deceased are a fit for their patients. The surgeons recover the organs and fly back to Hannover.

4:00 am: Dr. Strüber.'s cell rings: "We are ready."

4:40 am: A 52-year-old man is getting prepped to receive the heart of the deceased donor.

[...]

9:00 am: The heart transplant recipient is moved to ICU. Everything worked as planned. The surgeons continue working. They transplant the lungs into a 23-year-old, female patient. Later, a different team of surgeons transplants the liver into the same patient.

My donor had died in a traffic accident, and he saved two people when his life had been lost. In Germany, every organ donation is and must stay anonymous. I would have never found out anything about my donor if it wasn't for this article. I always knew I'd get my organs from a deceased donor, from someone who had died before their time, but this article made it even more real. My donor had been a person. Someone who had been on the road just around Christmas, driving to friends, home, who knew, and now he wasn't anymore. A fact so hard to grasp.

> **January 1, 2003, 2:52 p.m.**
> Everything's stable–anesthesia is slowly discontinued–next big hurdle, breathing independently.

My life still felt weird, and I disconnected from it, but I was aware how everyone around me greeted each other with a joyous "Happy New Year!"

Happy New Year? For my life I couldn't remember what I had done on New Year's Eve. Had I been out with friends? Had we made fondue (as it was custom in Germany)? Had I celebrated at someone's place, or had I been with my parents?

The more I racked my brain, the more I realized I hadn't done anything special for New Year's Eve and had probably been home with my parents. I had probably spent my last day of 2002 with them, doing nothing, being bored, and therefore had forgotten all about it.

I had no idea I was in the hospital, in ICU, because I had finally gotten my transplant. My brain was still too drugged to care.

> **January 2, 2003, 4:00 p.m.**
> Inka starts to breathe with support. She reacts when talked to.

I was becoming more and more aware of my surroundings, of what was happening to me throughout the day, and what to fear throughout the day. And the one thing I quickly learned to fear the most were my daily X-rays. Yes, X-rays.

Every morning, a radiologist came to my bed, dragging a portable X-ray machine behind him. While I stayed in bed, he adjusted the long arm of the X-ray machine above my chest, moved around the corner, pressed a button, and voila, my chest X-ray was taken. Without my having to move a single muscle. It would have been great if it weren't for the metal plate that first had to be placed in between my back and the mattress under me.

The radiologist shoved the plate under me in one swift move, and I couldn't do anything to stop him. I couldn't talk yet, I still had the breathing tube down my throat, and I couldn't sit up to make it easier for both of us. I was that weak—I couldn't even lift my head off my pillow.

Once the plate was in place, I had to lay on it for about fifteen seconds. Fifteen seconds of pain.

Then, with another shove, just in the opposite direction, the plate was removed and I was left alone. Only the back pain stayed to hang around.

My back, I didn't know it then, was covered by a huge hematoma. From my shoulders all the way down to my tailbone, my whole back was purple and black. All of it. Not patches here and there, no; the whole back was one purple and black surface.

When my mom saw it first, she was shocked. How could this happen? What had happened? One of my nurses was able to explain.

"It's from the operation," she told my mom. "Inka had been lying on the hard operation table for about ten hours. Being as skinny as she is, her whole back got bruised. No fat on her bones to cushion anything."

No wonder I was constantly in pain while constantly lying on my back.

January 3, 2003, 3:38 p.m.
Inka breathed alone for twenty minutes. It's very hard for her. We need to be patient. She's on the right path. Doctor is content.

On January 3, the doctors removed for the first time my breathing tube and let me breathe on my own for twenty minutes. According to my mom, it was a horrible sight. I was struggling with each breath. I was sweating, the oxygen level in my blood dropped further with every minute that passed, until I had to be placed back on ventilation. After only twenty minutes of breathing on my own, my lungs had failed.

I wasn't awake for any of this. I did what I was told to do, but more on autopilot than anything else. Not being able to breathe didn't faze me, but it did my mom.

After I was taken care of, she reached out to one of the doctors. "So, what does all this mean? Does it mean the lungs aren't working as they should? What do we do now?"

The doctor looked at her, confused for a second, and only then realized how my mom had never experienced anything like this before. She didn't know of the common complications after a lung transplant like the one they had just experienced.

"The lungs are working perfectly." He placed a calming hand on her arm. "Everything is working as it should."

"But why isn't she breathing?" my mom interrupted, not sure yet if she could trust his calm demeanor. I was put back on the ventilator. How could that be good?

"Inka can't breathe yet on her own because she has lost all her breathing muscles," the doctor explained. "She had lost so much weight after the transplant, her body consumed muscle instead of fat, including her breathing muscles. For her to be able to breathe on her own again, she has to build up these muscles again. And in order to do that, we will perform a tracheotomy tomorrow. This way we can supply her with extra oxygen *and* let her breathe on her own. It's not going to be easy for Inka, but it's going to work."

My mom had no further questions, but she had to sit down. Her legs had turned to jelly for a moment. Never had she imagined that the time after the transplant would be as fearful and as uncertain as the time before. For her, it felt like she still had a miles-long mine field she had to conquer before she could relax. Before she could say her daughter had made it.

My mom knew what a tracheotomy was. She had worked long enough as a doctor's assistant to know her way around common medical terms and procedures. A tracheotomy described a cut in the windpipe where a small tube would be inserted. Ventilation could be plugged on or plugged off from that tube. Either supply the patient with extra oxygen, or let the patient breathe on their own.

It made sense why the doctors decided on this route, but a small amount of fear still stayed behind. Another surgical intervention. Another anesthesia. Another day where my mom would sit and wait for my return from the operation room without knowing if everything was okay until she was able to see me.

Another day of fear.

17

Standing

The tracheotomy was done the following day around noon. It was a small procedure. My mom did not have to wait long before she was called back to sit by my side while I was waking up from the anesthesia. One of my former CF doctors, from the time before my transplant, had performed the tracheotomy, and my mom enjoyed talking to a familiar face while waiting for me to be conscious again. Though I was conscious. Or was I? I don't know, but I did wonder where I was and what had happened.

To me, it felt like I was lying in a white tiled room. I could hear my mom talking in the background. Something about if she could already come see me.

And suddenly I knew what had happened. My mom, and the doctor she spoke to, thought I was dead. Thought that I had died, and my mom wanted to come inside to say her final goodbyes to me.

I tried everything I could to move or say something, *anything* to let my mom know I wasn't dead, but it didn't work. Before I could tell her I was still alive, I was back asleep again.

I was brought up to ICU again where my sister was waiting for us. My mom needed some moral support, someone to lean on, someone to carry part of the burden together with her, and my sister had jumped in her car to be there for her.

"I'm going to go eat something," she told my sister once I was taken care of, and left. It was only the two of us, my sister and me, in my now private room in ICU.

My sister massaged my feet while I was waking up more and more from my anesthesia. I still couldn't talk—it required lots of practice to be able to talk with a hole punched through your windpipe—but my sister kept me entertained. She told me how my dog was doing, what she had been doing, all the unimportant things of everyday life outside the hospital. It was great until I realized I was hungry.

My sister told the nurse I was hungry but also mentioned how she thought I wasn't able to eat anything yet. I was still completely drunk, barely able to look straight, but the yogurt the nurse brought to my room I spooned in no time. Without choking or spilling any of it. My sister was impressed, and I went back to sleep.

The next time I woke up, my mom was back at my bedside, my sister on her way home, and I wrote on a piece of paper how I had already eaten a banana. I did not remember the yogurt, or my sister being there at all.

With the tracheotomy in place, I would be able to build up my breathing muscles again and even breathe on my own sooner than later. No obstacle in my way, except myself.

Because breathing had been such an exertion the whole time I had been in ICU, I was still under the assumption I had not been transplanted yet. Or at least not the lungs. How could I have gotten new lungs when breathing was still such a struggle? I was sure I had only gotten a new liver, and because I wasn't able to communicate and was drugged most of the time, no one explained anything to me.

I knew I had gotten a tracheotomy, but I didn't know why. I didn't know what was happening with me most of the time, and when one of the nurses came by and unplugged my tracheotomy (to have me breathe on my own), I freaked out. My eyes grew wide, and my arms reached for her, trying to grab her attention and make her listen to what I had to say. *"I have a lung disease! I can't breathe on my own. I need oxygen, or I will die."* But I couldn't say a single word. I felt like screaming under water for help while everyone watched from above the surface, as mute as myself.

I pointed for her to give me a piece of paper and wrote on it the name of my old CF doctor, the one who had performed the tracheotomy. Her name I knew, and I knew if the nurse would call her, she could explain why I needed oxygen and wasn't supposed to be unplugged under any circumstances.

I gave the paper back to my nurse, my stomach a painful knot of fear and helplessness, but of course she didn't know my old CF doctor. She only knew the doctors in ICU.

"Sorry," she said slowly, shaking her head at the paper, "I don't know this doctor, but everything is okay. Just keep breathing."

The phone rang, and my nurse left to pick up.

I just lay there. Terrified, helpless. I knew I only had to survive until my mom was back. My mom would tell her to plug the oxygen back in. My mom would save me. I only had to hold on. I had to keep breathing however possible and just stay alive.

The nurse looked around the corner, phone still pressed to her ear, and told me with a huge smile on her face, "I got your doctor on the line. He's very proud of you for breathing all by yourself. He said you should do five extra minutes. You are doing great."

Maybe it was good I wasn't able to speak. The F-word would've graced every sentence of mine, I'm sure.

Eventually, the five extra minutes of breathing were done, and I was reconnected with my oxygen supply. I had been breathing on my own for ten minutes and was drenched in sweat. I was utterly exhausted and shocked by the knowledge that even in ICU I had to fight for my life with everything I got.

Reconnected with the ventilation, it took me a moment to adjust *my* breathing rhythm with the one the machine had set for itself. I had to breathe in when the machine made me breathe in. Even my every breath wasn't under my control.

When my mom came back from her lunch, I tried to explain to her what had happened, but most of it got lost in translation. My handwriting was often undecipherable due to the constant trembling of my hands. The doctors said it was a side effect of all the medications I was still pumped with. Most of the time I was too drugged to make much sense. Like now, my mom had no idea what I was trying to tell her by writing *trying to kill me*, *lung disease*, and *stupid nurse* on a piece of paper.

Like so often, she just nodded along and told me she would talk to the nurses and/or the doctors about whatever I was talking about and got me off topic. I ate another yogurt, and another nurse came by and took a picture of me lying in my bed, smiling, pretending I had the best time ever.

And then I got the visitor who changed everything.

He entered my room like he owned it. Tall, wearing a white doctor's coat, he marched right up to my bed, reached out his hand, and introduced himself.

"Hello. I'm the doctor who picked up the lungs and liver for you and flew them back to Hannover. How are you doing?"

And that's when it finally clicked. I had gotten lungs and a liver. I had truly gotten lungs *and* a liver! I couldn't believe it. Suddenly everything made sense. Suddenly everything was nothing but amazing.

I held up my right thumb to answer his question and smiled like an idiot.

"Good." His eyes landed on my nurse, who had just come in to bring me another huge bag of IV medications.

"Is there any chance," he asked her, "to unplug Inka from her tubes and have her stand up?"

The nurse was as surprised as I was.

"Do you want to stand up?" she asked me, and I nodded. I wasn't sure at all if I wanted to stand up, or even could stand up, as I still wasn't able to lift my head or sit up on my own, but sure, I'd stand up. I had gotten a new set of lungs and a liver. I could do anything. I was ready to do a cartwheel if the doctor asked me to.

"Then, let's do it," the nurse said, now again talking to the tall doctor. With his help, she unplugged all the tubes I still had attached to my body. It took a while, but eventually I was free.

"First," my new favorite doctor said, "I'll have you sit on the edge of your bed, feet dangling over the edge. Nothing else, okay?"

I nodded and with his help, I sat up and slid my feet over the edge of my bed.

It was a weird feeling having no mattress pressed against my back. No support whatsoever. My head felt a little woozy, but it passed as I just sat there, ridiculous grin on my face, waiting for further instructions.

"Now," the doctor said, "you will stand up. I need you to lock your knees once you're up, otherwise you won't be able to hold your weight. You can use my coat to pull yourself up if you need to. Ready?"

I nodded and then did exactly what he had suggested. I grabbed his coat with both hands and pulled myself up.

He flinched for a second, followed by a bark of laughter and an honest "Wow!"

In my head, I screamed "Hell yes!" and was up. I was fucking standing. I had a new lung and a new liver. And I was standing.

"You are taller than I thought you were," my nurse said, standing at least half a head shorter than me.

"Right," the doctor agreed. "You looked so tiny lying in bed. I'm surprised too."

I didn't stand long. It was a very wobbly business. Like when Bambi took his first steps, but it felt so good having a short taste of what normal life could be like. For a week, I hadn't been able to do anything but lie on my back. I wasn't able to turn to my side, I wasn't able to sit up, lift my head, or just scratch my ass. Now standing, even if it was only for a short moment, I felt like I was on top of the world.

When the tall doctor left and I was back in bed, reconnected to the countless tubes around me, I took a piece of paper and a pen from my mom and wrote in spidery words: *What the fuck, I already have new lungs!* Followed by two huge smiley faces.

> **January 5, 2003, 12:46 p.m.**
> Pure gratitude! To donor and doctors! Inka is doing fine. She sat in a chair today. She smiles. She's breathing with less and less support.

The following days were filled with determination. Finally, I had a direction to go to, a goal to reach, a purpose. In addition, my head and my thoughts got clearer every day. I was even able to realize how all my dreams about evil nurses, my sister showering other patients, and doctors harvesting organs right beside me had not been real. Only the dreams with Ingo in them, that I was sure about, had been real though he didn't come to visit anymore. I missed him. Missed writing letters to him, but my hand coordination wasn't good enough yet, to attempt to write one. I only exchanged notes with my mom. She talked, I wrote short answers, and when we were out of words, we played board games.

It was during a game of Yahtzee that we first realized something was wrong. Every time I tried to flip the dice cup with my left hand, I spilled the dice instead. Somehow, I couldn't flip the cup properly. My arm just wouldn't listen to me.

Once my mom brought my laptop to the hospital, I realized I also had coordination problems while typing. Though still only with my left hand.

We talked to the doctors, but they were as clueless as we were.

"Give it time," was the overall suggestion and with a shrug, we filed it as *not important* and moved on with our boring hospital lives.

> **January 7, 2003, 1:43 p.m.**
> Everything is slowly getting better. Inka sits in her chair and even ate lunch. Breathing is improving. She glows!

Three days later, my breathing had improved so much, I was now able to breathe a whole day on my own. The doctors said I was ready to have my tracheotomy removed.

At first, I was super excited. Without the tracheotomy in my throat, I would finally be able to talk. It had been so long since I had been able to speak my mind. Thirteen days. I couldn't wait! Finally, I would be able to ask any question I had, say what I wanted and what I didn't want, and pester the nurses until I got answers.

Of course, I had written down many questions during the last days, but almost never had I gotten a satisfying answer. The ICU nurses simply didn't have the time to stand beside my bed, wait for me to scribble everything down, and then answer it. It was impossible to have a real conversation this way, but once I'd get my voice back . . . may God have mercy on their souls. I'd ask them *everything*.

The removal of the tracheotomy was easy. One quick pull, a huge Band-Aid was placed over the hole in my throat, and that was it. The hole would eventually close on its own. Normally within a few days.

My doctor, my ICU nurse, and my mom stood around my bed and stared at me in eager anticipation for me to say my first words after almost two weeks of silence.

But before I said anything, I looked at my oxygen saturation. Was I breathing okay? Was I ready to be taken off any kind of ventilation?

It was at 96 percent.

"Your breathing is perfect," my doctor reassured me. "Anything above ninety-five percent is perfect. No need to worry. Your lungs are doing what they're supposed to do. How does it feel to breathe finally on your own?"

"It feels scary."

My mom and I looked up in surprise. My voice was . . . different. It sounded scratchy, and it sounded breathless. As if I wasn't able to say two words in a row without sucking in air in between. As if I had just run up a hill and was still catching my breath while telling a story.

"Is that normal?" My mom pointed at me, not saying anything else, but my doctor understood immediately what she meant.

"Yes," he said. "It will take her some time to talk and breathe normally. Eventually, it'll all sync itself. It just needs some time."

"I'll come in every half hour to check your oxygen saturation," the nurse said and with that, my mom and I were left alone.

"This is weird," I said when the door closed behind them. "I sound so weird. And it feels so weird not having any ventilation anymore." I felt hot, sweaty, and as if my chest were tightening.

I glanced again over my shoulder at my oxygen level.

"It's at ninety-five percent," my mom said.

I nodded. Everything was good. The tight chest was probably just my nerves playing tricks on me. No reason to worry, but I couldn't help myself. "What if I get tired at some point and can't breathe anymore? What will they do then? Reintubate me? Put me back on ventilation?"

"You won't get tired," my mom said matter-of-factly. "You were breathing on your own all day yesterday. And you are in ICU. Nothing will happen to you here. They know what they're doing. They will keep you safe no matter what."

I knew my mom was right. Even if I got tired and couldn't breathe anymore on my own, they wouldn't just let me die. Worst case, they would reintubate me, put me back on ventilation, and then reevaluate; but still, I couldn't shake the fear of running out of breath.

My mom and I talked the whole afternoon. About everything. How my dad was doing, how it felt to live with my aunt and her family during this time, the newspaper article of my donor. I also watched my mom send another text to everyone, saying:

January 10, 2003, 1:35 p.m.
Inka is breathing by herself! We are all overly happy.
The miracle is perfect! Endless gratitude!

I listened to her read the many responses that kept coming in afterward and still, my mind always found its way back to the one question I couldn't let go of: What if my lungs suddenly stopped breathing?

When my mom was ready to drive back home to my aunt's house for the night, I had accumulated so much fear that I was close to hysteria.

The whole day I had breathed and breathed and breathed. My oxygen saturation had never dropped below ninety-five percent. There was no reason whatsoever that my lungs couldn't keep breathing through the night . . . but still, I was terrified to be left alone. I was terrified of dying, of suffocating, of having no one around to save me.

"I want to speak to a psychologist," I told my mom, my nurse, and even the doctor who came in for a short moment to hear what was going on. But it was already too late for a psychologist.

"It's now 7:36 p.m.," my doctor said, looking at his watch. "Every psychologist is home by now. We won't get any of them here before tomorrow morning."

"Then you have to stay here," I said to my mom, reaching out my hand so I could cling to her and never let go. "You have to stay here and make sure I won't stop breathing."

My mom looked at my outstretched hand, gave a curt shake with her head, and placed her hands on her hips, ready to tackle this problem once and for all.

"I won't stay here all night and watch you breathe," she said loud and clear. "This is crazy. You are in ICU. Every alarm will sound if you stop breathing. I can't just sit here all night."

It sounded harsh, but the still-rational part of my brain agreed with her. All this time we had kept our heads on straight. Not once had we become hysterical when bad news arrived. Because this was our strength. Be rational and just dealing with it. Nurturing my fear to suffocate wasn't part of it. I had to keep a clear mind to make it through this. This was an obstacle I had to tackle by myself, and I would because my mom was there to make sure of it.

"Let's do it like this instead," my doctor chimed in, putting all his white-coat-wearing-authority into his words. "Your mom will drive home now. You will rest a little bit, and before *I* drive home, I promise you I will stop by and see how you're doing."

"Promise?" I asked.

"Promise," he said, and he did.

It was around 9:00 p.m. when he came back to see me.

He pulled a chair close and sat down beside my bed. "Tell me what's the problem."

I didn't have anything new to tell him. My fears were still the same as they had been a few hours ago. Same as he couldn't tell me anything new either. My lungs were still breathing fine. My oxygen saturation was still great—nothing had changed. But having my doctor sit beside my bed at 9:00 p.m., knowing that all he wanted to do was drive home and spend time with his family, made all the difference. He still came to reassure me that I was *not* going to die tonight.

I was so grateful for his attention. And I was so grateful for him acknowledging what I had been through. Of course, my fear was irrational, but having your lungs exchanged was just as irrational. He didn't judge me. He just sat there, talked, listened; eventually, I was ready to trust him (*and* my new lungs) and was able to say good night to him.

I survived the night without any complications. When I woke up, the real horror started.

18

Goddamn Yogurt

"Good morning!" my nurse cheered the moment she came into my room. "Today you'll do most of the morning chores yourself since you're finally breathing all on your own. We'll start with getting you out of bed so you can brush your teeth at the sink and not in bed anymore."

And that's how it continued throughout the whole day. Off my ventilation, I wasn't allowed to sit in bed anymore and let everyone around me take care of everything. All of a sudden, I had to do most of it myself. Brushing my teeth, combing my hair, getting dressed, sitting in a chair for breakfast, not staying in bed anymore. My bed was from now on reserved for sleeping only.

Truly a nightmare.

When my mom came in, I was sitting in my chair, still munching on my breakfast, and already exhausted beyond belief. Everything I did required a huge amount of energy I didn't have. Not only my breathing muscles had withered away during the last two weeks, but every other muscle was also gone. Lifting my toothbrush and brushing my teeth felt like I was training for the Olympics weightlifting team. Walking from my bed to the sink and back felt like marathon training, and brushing my hair was almost impossible. But if I ever wanted to leave this godforsaken place, I had to get back on my feet. I was already able to lift my head by myself, but still too weak to get out of bed without help.

I still had a long way ahead of me.

In the afternoon, a physiotherapist came to see me. Apparently, news had spread that I was mobile and could be kicked out of bed at any given time.

I was told to lift my arms, use my feet to push away the physiotherapist's hands, walk rounds in my tiny room, and stretch.

"You look very skinny," my physiotherapist said, "but you still have quite a good amount of strength." And that was the last time I ever saw her.

She never stopped by again. From that moment on, it was up to my mom and me to get me back on my feet. Naturally, my mom didn't waste any time. The physiotherapist was gone, and my mom was ready to go shopping.

"Let's go downstairs to the shopping street. Come on. It'll be good for you to see something else besides this room," she said over and over again because I absolutely didn't want to go.

When my mom brought my nurse to my room for reinforcement, I knew I had lost the battle. Together with the help of my nurse, my mom placed me into one of the hospital's wheelchairs (I wasn't able yet to go down by myself) and together we went downstairs. Shopping for yogurt when I could get it from one of my nurses. I hated it and let it show all the way.

But when the nurse wheeled me inside the kiosk downstairs and I picked out a yogurt my mom could buy for me, her smile made me forget any anger. She was so excited to see me participate in life again, choosing a goddamn yogurt, that it made every effort worth it.

When I was back in my room, I went back to bed and fell asleep. My first day without ventilation had been horrible, but also a huge success.

In the evenings, I still got a high-calorie drink flushed down my feeding tube. It was always the last thing my nurse did before the night nurse took over, and today was no different.

I was lying on my back in my bed, sheets fresh, night gown clean, teeth brushed, and my hair put neatly together. I watched my nurse flush the high-calorie drink down through some kind of a funnel. I burped a little. I could taste the nasty drink but tried to concentrate on *not* paying attention to it. It would be over soon. The bottle was almost empty. Almost all that nasty drink was inside of my stomach, no need to burp again. But then my nurse had the brilliant idea to rinse it all down with sparkling water, and I couldn't hold myself anymore.

With one huge barf, it all came back up. And because I still wasn't able to sit up without help, I barfed it all out while lying flat on my back. It was just wonderful.

When everything was cleaned again—me, my hair, my teeth, my bedsheets, my night gown—the feeding tube was pulled as well. No more funneled high-calorie drinks from now on.

If I had known, I would have barfed a long time ago.

January 12, 2003, 10:13 p.m.
Medical parameters look great. Inka has problems with her back. She's not sleeping well. These days are excruciatingly hard for her.

On January 13, I was moved from the ICU to a so-called stepdown room, a half ICU, and it was a relief. I was still observed closely but not 24/7 anymore as in ICU. A nurse poked her head in occasionally, asked if everything was good, but that was all. This also marked the time when I was responsible for all my medications again. None of my meds were administered via IV anymore, as all of them were pills. I had to make sure I took the right amount of them every day.

It felt great getting some self-responsibility back. I had been treated like a child throughout the whole last three weeks because I hadn't been able to do anything myself; I hadn't been able to talk and, due to the constant sedation, hadn't even been allowed to make any decisions. Being entrusted with taking care of my own meds felt amazing. And to push my independence even further along, I also got some kind of a rope ladder attached to the foot of my bed. With the help of this ladder, I was finally able to get myself out of bed after lying down. Without any help.

Slowly, slowly, I was becoming a fully functional human being again and could feel the Inka I had once been start to emerge. I joked around a lot with my mom, with the nurses and doctors too; I missed my friends as well. After so many months of actively avoiding them, I now felt desperate to talk to them—anyone beside my mom and/or medical personnel. Which is why my mom's next text read:

> **January 16, 2003, 12:14 p.m.**
> Inka is getting bored! Letters can be sent to the following address of her aunt . . .

Everybody wrote me a letter, an actual letter, no email. Close friends, acquaintances, fellow students, even some friends of friends who just felt the need to congratulate me as well. It was wonderful. It didn't take long, and every empty surface of my room was stacked with congratulation cards. Finally, some color in my otherwise white/beige/grayish room.

> **January 17, 2003, 3:01 p.m.**
> It is unbelievable! Inka is walking down the hall! The doctors are very content! Inka is impatient. She still has a long way to go.

It was almost three weeks past my transplant, and still no physiotherapist had found her way back to my room, which is why my never-too-tired-to-walk mom and I took my recovery into our own hands. We walked. Everywhere. All the time never ending. At first, we took a wheelchair with us, just in case, but it didn't take long for my mom to decide I didn't need one.

"No one gains back their strength by sitting in a chair," she said wherever I dared to complain. "Let's continue walking, shall we?"

A few times I considered pushing her down the stairs. I also wasn't allowed to take the elevator anymore, but since she was the only one who bought me a Hawaii toast without Hawaii every afternoon, I refrained from it. Also, she was the only company I had and company I needed. Being able to chat and joke with my mom every day was the one thing that kept me going. Figuratively and literally.

After every one of our endless walks, we would sit downstairs on one of the chairs alongside the shopping street and I would eat my non-Hawaii Hawaii toast while my mom drank coffee; we'd watched the same doctors and nurses walk by every day. Until one day my mom decided to turn our observations into a dating market.

"Do you prefer a doctor or a nurse?" she asked out of the blue.

I looked up from my toast. "What do you mean? In case I get hit by a bus? Definitely a doctor."

"I mean as a boyfriend. What else?"

"As a boyfriend?" A boyfriend was the last thing on my mind, but okay.

I watched some nurses and two doctors pass by. None looked interesting. Not even for my low standards after being locked inside a hospital for weeks, but I was ready for any crazy idea my mom could come up with to keep boredom away.

"Nurse," I eventually said. "A doctor will tell me all the time what to do and what not to do and when to take my medications, to check my blood sugar and whatnot. Unless"—I raised my finger—"he's extremely good-looking. Then I might make an exception."

"Our main selection criterion is good looks?" My mom raised her eyebrows at me. "Ever heard of the phrase 'Those who live in glass houses shouldn't throw stones'?"

I couldn't help but laugh. She had a point. I looked like a walking dead person. Still extremely skinny, tubes sticking out of my body, not to mention the scars covering my body. The longest being thirteen inches.

"In my case," I said, sitting up straight and proud, looking at my mom, "it's my inner values a man will be rewarded with. If you can get a woman like me, who cares about a few scars."

"Point well made," my mom said, nudging me. "Good-looking it is."

We kept looking, commenting, and even took a few patients into consideration, but no one seemed right. Eventually, getting tired of this game, my mom said, "Okay, the next one coming around the corner, exiting the elevators, will be it. We will leave it up to fate.

Whoever comes around the corner next will be your match and you will have to introduce yourself to him."

"Okay," I said, and we both stared in the direction of the elevators, curious who fate would come up with.

After only a few seconds, we could hear the elevator ping to a halt on our floor. Voices drifted toward us from people exiting and boarding the arrived elevator, and then a man turned the corner, leaving us both speechless.

He looked like a hippy nurse. Long, messy hair. Here and there a colorful extension weaved into it, slouching past us while blowing bubblegum.

Instead of jumping up and talking to my future husband, we both burst out laughing. Of all the people we had watched go by during the last hour, of all the people we had considered during the last hour, this one stood out. Fate was right. I didn't need good looks, I needed different.

After we were able to look at each other again without laughing, my future boyfriend was long gone. I had missed my opportunity to meet the man fate had chosen for me, but it was okay. I laughed like I hadn't laughed in a very long time. Laughing without coughing was just the best.

These silly moments, in which we laughed about the most stupid things, were the ones that kept me alive. Everything else in my life was still life-or-death serious. On the outside, it might have seemed as if I were out of the woods. My lungs were breathing, my liver was filtering, everything worked. But at the same time, everything was still balancing on a thin wire over a chasm. Nothing was taken lightly, which is why Mom and I needed to relax from time to time and simply laugh. Because so far, there was nothing else to laugh about.

When we came back to my room after finding the "man of my dreams," my mom went to get herself another coffee and I grabbed my phone, for the first time since my transplant, and called Martina.

While I was talking to Martina, my mom stood outside my door, coffee forgotten in her hand, and watched me connecting with the outside world for the first time since my transplant. There in the doorframe of my room, she cried.

In the evening, Dr. N., the man who had transplanted my liver, came to see me. I had just finished my dinner, sitting comfortably in my bed, when he entered. He greeted my mom and immediately asked, "Why are you in bed? It's six thirty. You shouldn't be in bed, you should be outside, walking around."

Another person who was obsessed with walking.

"I already did walk today," I said. "My mom is—"

But he didn't really listen. He found my dinner tray and lifted the cover.

"Why didn't you finish your dinner?" he asked and turned back to look at me.

"Eh . . . because the food at the hospital is not good?" I asked, not sure what was expected of me. I mean, I was recovering from a lung *and* liver transplant. One wasn't allowed to rest past six after surviving such an operation?

"You could order pizza if you don't like the food," he suggested, leaving my mom and I completely dumbstruck.

Pizza? Pizza was such an ordinary thing; I couldn't imagine myself eating pizza only three weeks after my transplant. Pizza was something for healthy folks. For all the people who sat in front of their TV right now, Bud Light in hand, feet on an ottoman. I did not feel like pizza could be part of my new life yet. My mom obviously felt the same.

"You can have pizza delivered to a hospital?" she asked.

"Sure," Dr. N said. "The nurses do it all the time. Just ask them, and they'll tell you where to call."

We never ordered pizza while we were at the hospital, and I was not allowed to be in bed before 7:00 p.m. anymore, but I did fall out of bed once because I reached for the lame hospital dinner standing too far away on my nightstand one evening.

I missed the nightstand by a hair, fell headfirst out of my bed, and banged my shoulder. I was lucky I didn't rip out my liver drainage on my way down. The bag for the drainage was normally attached to a hock under my bed, but that evening it had been lying on my blanket. Thank God.

Before I could eat the lame dinner I had so desperately reached for, I had to get an X-ray to make sure I didn't break anything. The next morning, my doctors suggested calling the children's department to ask for some side rails for my bed so I wouldn't fall out again. Now it was their time to have a good laugh, and they weren't too shy to make use of it.

The liver drainage was pulled a few days later. A surgeon I hadn't met before came to my room and pulled it out. No sedation, no hesitation, just one inch at a time. The drainage was eight inches long.

It wasn't painful, but it was one of the weirdest feelings ever. I could feel the drainage being pulled out of my abdomen; I watched it grow longer and longer while my surgeon made small talk with my mom. That's why surgeons should only be allowed around sedated patients. They lack empathy. All of them. Most of them. Or at least some of them.

January 31, 2003, 9:38 a.m. (text from me)
I'm still sitting in snow-white Hannover, but tomorrow we'll drive to snow-white Dalheim, home. Finally! Kiss, Inka

My last evening in Hannover. Tomorrow, my mom and I would drive home. I couldn't wait. I couldn't believe it. I couldn't sleep. I was still up at around 8:00 p.m., late for a hospital evening, when someone knocked on my door.

"Yes," I yelled. Probably the night nurse, wanting to ask me why I wasn't in bed yet, but it was another patient. A young woman, maybe a few years younger than me, who poked her head in.

"Hi," she said, somehow apologetic, standing in my doorframe. She was as skinny as I, shoulders pulled up to assist her breathing—for sure CF as well. Her hair was pulled together into a messy ponytail. "I've asked the nurse if I can come by, if I'm allowed to come see you. You know, because of germs and viruses and all of that," she explained, and I nodded.

"Anyway," she continued, "the nurse had said it's okay as long as I wear a mask." She pointed at her face mask, and I nodded again. I still had no clue why she was here in my room, on my last day.

"I came by because I know you're already post-transplant and I'm still waiting for mine and was wondering if I could maybe ask you a few questions about your experience."

Ah, finally, it all made sense.

"Sure," I said and waved her inside. "What do you wanna know?"

We didn't talk for long. She was as exhausted as I had been before my transplant. Immediately out of breath, and the mask didn't help either. But I answered most of her questions and, most important, was able to give her hope. She was waiting as a high urgency patient and was, same as I had been, desperate to get it over with.

She made it to her transplant but died on the operating table due to heart failure. Barely twenty-two years old.

I only heard about this weeks later during one of our checkup visits in Hannover, but it stuck with me. The whole story stuck with me. It reminded me how lucky I had been to have survived my transplant. It could have gone any other way. An organ transplant was still the only and best chance, especially for patients with CF, to extend their lifetime, but it wasn't a guarantee. Not at all. It was more like Russian roulette. Some made it, some didn't. And the ones who didn't I never forgot.

19

Life 2.0

Every time my mom left my hospital room by the end of the day, waved a goodbye, and blew a kiss in my direction, I wished nothing more than for her to be the one with IVs stuck inside her arms and nasty hospital food for dinner. *I* wanted to leave the hospital. *I* wanted to wave an arrogant goodbye, blow a kiss, and stroll out of there with glee and drive to my aunt's place. But then, eventually, the day came.

I was allowed to leave. To leave for good. I was so happy, I wanted to dissolve into tears, but in the end, I only waved and smiled. Waved and smiled.

> **February 1, 2003, 10:29 a.m.**
> We are incredibly happy! We can go home! Kisses to all of you!

It was an incredible feeling sitting in my mom's car, driving on the Autobahn, seeing the snow-covered landscape fly by, and getting closer and closer to be able to hug my dad again. To drive down their neighborhood, seeing their house, opening their front door, and falling into his arms. It had only been thirty-six days since I had seen my dad's face grow smaller and smaller as we started our journey toward Hannover, wondering if I would ever see him again. And now I would. It was an incredible feeling. To have survived.

To still be here.

To be home.

Only one more person I had to tell all about it:

> Dear Ingo,
>
> You won't believe it, since today I'm back home at my parents' place, including new organs! It was an extremely hard time, but somehow I made it. Well, I'm sure you know what I'm talking about—you were by my side many times. Thank you for that!
>
> Normally, I should have been in rehab by now, but since I walked a million steps at the hospital without having a professional force me to, the doctors decided to let me take care of my own rehab. I can do everything from home, just like before my transplant, and am very happy about it. Home.
>
> But I have to say, coming home, finally starting life 2.0, it feels different than I imagined. My new life has started, but I'm not able to feel it yet. Most of the time, I don't even know what to feel. I don't feel sick anymore, but I also don't feel healthy. I feel empty. I imagined my new life grand, colorful, and exciting, and now I can't even say with certainty if it's started or not, or where I am right now.

Am I ungrateful when I think like that? When I can't burst with gratitude? Am I unrealistic if I wished the beginning of my new life to be filled with confetti parades and celebrating people in the streets?

Okay, you don't have to answer the last question, but yes, that's how I imagined it. But there are no parades inside of me, only emptiness and the feeling of being lost. How do I start my new life? I can't even imagine going back to university. Can't imagine anything right now. It feels as if I'm still standing with one foot in the hereafter, with the other one in life and under me is a huge chasm. I can't feel myself, don't know who Inka really is and where the old Inka, the one I knew so well, went. As if I must find myself all over again. — Your feeling-overjoyed-but-also-lost niece

Back home, my mom and I jumped right back into our routine. In some ways, it was different now; in other ways, it was the same shit as before my transplant. Every day we drove to physiotherapy, my mom forced me to take a walk with her and I'd call my friends here and there, but otherwise it still felt like I was waiting for something. Time was still ticking slowly. My body was still slow. Life was slow. As my mom had written in one of her texts from the hospital, everything was going too slow for me. I wanted to jump right back into life. I wanted to go from *waiting to die*, right back to *living at 120 mph*. I was ready, but my body wasn't, as it showed me very clearly on February 4, after we had been home for only four days.

The night had been good, but when I sat at the breakfast table that Tuesday morning, nothing felt right.

"I don't know." I pushed my plate farther away from me. "I'm not really hungry."

"Maybe an egg?" my dad asked, but I shook my head.

"Coffee at least?" My mom joined in, but even coffee made me cringe.

"I think I'll go back to bed," I said and stood up. Two worried pairs of eyes followed me. I was worried too. There was no reason why I should feel bad. I was able to breathe. My liver was doing what a liver should be doing, and still, something seemed wrong.

I went back to bed hoping whatever was wrong would solve itself by sleep and rest. The whole day I spent in my room, watched TV, napped, but nothing helped.

And then the twitching started.

It started in my lower left arm. Like a triggered nerve that was twitching, only from time to time. On the same arm that had caused me problems while typing on a keyboard or flipping a dice cup back in the ICU.

The words of my doctors in Hannover came back to my mind: *"Give it time."* And I did. All day I rested my arm, propped it up on a pillow, massaged it when it twitched again, but nothing helped. By the evening, the twitching had only spread. Now, when twitching, it went up all the way to my neck. It was weird and frightening, but none of us could come up with a reason for it. Only my nausea we could treat, and that's what we concentrated on.

My mom drove to the pharmacy and got me a strong anti-nausea medication. Something chemotherapy patients took.

I immediately swallowed one of the pills once my mom was back, and then we all sat in front of the TV, waiting for a miracle recovery, but instead the twitching came back with a vengeance. This time it went all the way up to my eyebrow. We collectively freaked out. My mom went white and ran into the kitchen to get the info sheet of the anti-nausea medication I had just swallowed.

"It might be, my God, it might be an allergic reaction!" she yelled from the kitchen. Her voice was high and pitchy, unnatural.

"I'll call an ambulance." My dad reached with jerky movements for the phone while I just stared at the TV without seeing anything, only concentrating on my twitching and willing it with everything I had to stop. This couldn't be happening. This just couldn't be real.

When the EMTs finally arrived, the twitching was gone again, but I still decided to go to the hospital. Something was wrong, no matter how much I wanted to will it away.

The EMTs were the same ones that had driven me to the airport in Düsseldorf on the day of my transplant. They were very excited to see me now, transplanted and breathing again.

All the way to the hospital, I chatted with the one in the back, and my mom got the one in the front seat up to date.

When we arrived at the hospital, I almost felt like I shouldn't have come at all. The twitching hadn't returned, my vitals were all perfect, and my nausea was gone due to the medication my mom had given me. I was in a good mood after a fun drive to the hospital, but my mom put her foot down.

"We stay here," she said, resolute. "Someone has to figure out why you don't feel well and where the twitching is coming from. Before we don't know what's going on, I won't take you back home."

Well then.

The doctor at the ER thought the same. He didn't know what to make of my symptoms, but he strongly agreed with my mother to observe me during the night. I wasn't convinced.

"Why should I stay when I feel fine now?" I asked my mom a hundred times, but she didn't budge.

"Because something is wrong with you," she answered a hundred times back. "Or do you think it's normal to feel nauseous all day and have weird twitching along your arm, all the way up to your eyebrow?"

"It hasn't twitched for a while now." I shrugged. "Maybe it's gone." Though we both knew it wasn't. And the moment one of the doctors came in to see me inside the room they had assigned to me, I got proof that it wasn't gone. It was back.

"It's twitching again," I told the doctor and pointed at my arm. "All the way up to my eyebrow, and it's starting to be painful."

It wasn't simple twitching anymore; it felt more like a spasm.

"It's painful," I said again, this time with fear in my voice. "And it's moving up to my neck too."

"Breathe," my mom said from behind the doctor. "Try to relax, don't panic."

I could see the white all around her irises and knew panic was the only emotion available.

I wanted to tell her there was no way I could calm down when suddenly everything cramped up, my head bent sideways, and I passed out.

My whole body was cramping. Foam spilled out of my mouth. I wasn't breathing and started to turn blue.

"Help!" my mom yelled and ran out of my room, leaving the doctor behind. He didn't know what to do. He froze. "Help!" she yelled down the hall. Within seconds, nurses and another doctor came running.

My mom stepped aside, slid down the wall, and sat on the floor. Her hands were shaking when she called my dad.

"You need to come to the hospital," she said the moment Dad picked up. "Inka just had a seizure."

20

Mushroom Farm

When my dad arrived, I was already awake again, sitting in a bed in ICU, joking and having a good time. The seizure had stopped by itself. My lungs didn't get damaged. I didn't bite my tongue; all was good except for one question: Where did that seizure come from?

Hannover was called, but they had no idea either. My transplant doctors suggested I'd stay in ICU for a few days to see if I had any more seizures. Once released, we had to find out what had caused all this. My left arm not being able to flip the dice cup wasn't something benign anymore. From one moment to another, it became topic number one. No one talked about my new lungs and liver anymore—everything was about my seizure and my weird left arm.

This was serious.

I stayed for four days in the hospital, but nothing happened. I didn't have another seizure, I didn't feel sick anymore, I was fine.

Many speculations were phrased during these four days, but no one knew for sure what was wrong. Instead of guessing, Hannover sent over a list of tests I had to do once I was released. A CT of my head, an EEG to measure the electric activity of my brain, an ultrasound of my heart, and an ENG to measure nerve conduction velocity.

It was absolutely sickening.

Dear Ingo,

Life is starting to take shape, even though it's not the shape I had dreamed of. Every week my mom and I drive to Hannover for a lung checkup. So far no one has dared to give an estimate when my time in between checkups will be increased. Besides driving to Hannover every week, I also have to do all these other tests to find out where my seizure came from. It feels almost like before my transplant, only now I can breathe while sitting at the doctors' offices waiting for appointments.

The seizure . . . I'm still digesting it. Same as my mom. She said seeing my seizure had cost her a nail to her coffin. God, I believe her. And now the constant fear of having another one. I didn't really experience the seizure, I passed out immediately, and still I'm scared of having another one. Weird, isn't it?

When I'm not complaining about doctor visits, I'm struggling to process everything that has happened to me during these last months. I mean the transplant. It's difficult to wrap my head around it. To digest the change from dying and now being thrown back into life.

Do you think there are feelings that don't really exist? That can't be described or grasped? That aren't even

> designed for the human mind to understand?
>
> That's how the magnitude of my transplant feels like. Just think about it, I stole life from death. Death became life. You think death agrees with this practice? That I'm still alive even though I was dying? Isn't that bad publicity? For death and life?
>
> But I also did something normal last week: I went out. With Silke! She picked me up, and we drove to a café where we met with another friend of hers. OMG, it was so nice. So nice being a normal, young adult. Only my strength is still lacking. I had to pull myself out of Silke's car; my legs weren't strong enough to just lift me out. Another reason why life still feels strange to me. I don't fit into it yet; it still is a struggle.
>
> Next week, I have all my seizure appointments, and at the beginning of March, we'll be, once again, in Hannover. Hopefully we will know by then what's wrong with my head. — Your still-more-in-hospitals-than-at-home niece

When my mom and I arrived in Hannover on March 3, we felt pretty good about how everything was going. My lungs and liver were doing great, and the results of my seizure tests all came back benign. Well, almost all of them. The CT of my head showed a small shadow on the right side of my head that didn't belong there, but it was tiny. Only a few millimeters big. The size of a lowercase o typed on a piece of paper. I wasn't concerned. Something that small couldn't be too dangerous.

It was my post-liver transplant doctor who set us straight and let hell rain down on us while we sat in her sterile, under-furnished office, trying to get comfortable on yet another set of plastic chairs, ready to talk about my well-working liver and the tiny shadow in my head.

"This is very bad," she said multiple times, oozing authority behind her meticulously organized desk, while reading the radiologist report over and over.

"Something is growing inside your head that doesn't belong there, that's most likely linked to your seizure, and now we need to find out as quickly as possible what it is that's growing there and what we can do to get rid of it."

"But it's so small." I tried one more time to ease the terror she was conjuring, but she just wouldn't let me put on rose-colored glasses.

"Two millimeters are not small when we're talking about a mass inside your brain," she said sternly. "We also don't know how fast it's growing. It could have been a millimeter last week. This is very, very serious, Inka. I'll call the neurology department right now and find a bed for you. You need to stay here until we figure this out."

"But . . ." I could feel tears coming, "I don't want to stay in the hospital. I don't even have clothes. I want to go back home, I . . ."

I looked at my mom, who was accompanying me as always, hoping for her to help me put some sense back into my doctor, but my mom had already realized this was serious. Horrifyingly serious.

"This"—my doctor cut me off and pointed at the report—"will kill you if we don't find a way to treat it. You will stay here, no questions asked. Your mom can get you clothes and everything else, but you have to stay here. This is not a joke, this"—she pointed once again at the report—"is fatal if we don't treat it, and not a reason to cry."

She stood up, grabbed the report, and left us alone. Probably to call the neurologists to let them know I was coming to be their new patient.

My mom put her hand on my arm. She was pale like the paper that stupid radiology report was printed on, but as always, she was ready to fight once again. "She's right," Mom said. "We have to take care of this. We can't risk another seizure. We can't ignore it."

"I know," I said and pulled up my nose. I wasn't crying because I had to stay at the hospital and didn't want to. I was crying because of everything else. Something was growing inside my head. Something that might kill me. Despite having new lungs and liver. How could anyone not cry facing this? I had just defeated death, and now he was after me again. And this time, it wasn't something I could fight by doing more exercise or eating more calories. This time, my life rested solely in the hands of modern medicine. Either my doctors and their medicine could save me, or I'd die.

I had nothing left to do but cry.

My mom drove toward home that evening and met my dad halfway at a rest stop. They exchanged clothes and a hug, then she came back to Hannover to stay with me. Again, Mom found shelter at her sister Renate's place. It almost felt like our weeks right after transplant. Once again killing time in Hannover's shopping street. Walking stairs and—this was new—having unfamiliar tests done.

First, Hannover did another EEG. The hospital in my parents' town did one too, but of course, Hannover had to do their own EEG. And to everyone's surprise, the EEG done in Hannover came back clean.

I had my nerve conduction velocity tested, and an ultrasound of my heart was done. Though this time the heart was scanned from the inside, from the feeding tube, and not from the outside. For this procedure, I had to swallow a tube, and because I wanted to be able to eat right after the procedure, I agreed to do it without sedation.

Never again.

The whole process only took about four minutes, but during the whole four minutes I gagged and suppressed the urge to just pull that darn tube out of my throat and slap the doctor in the face with it. An absolutely unnecessary experience.

My heart was normal, thank God, and I was set up to get an MRI of my head next. And finally, we found the reason for my seizure.

The reason I couldn't flip a dice cup with my left hand.

The reason I couldn't type on a keyboard.

I had a fungus growing inside my brain. Or a mushroom farm, as my sister and I would name it later.

The fungus—that was the guess of my doctors—had probably come from my old lungs. During my transplant, I had been hooked up to the heart-lung machine for a short amount of time. It had saved my life but had also disabled the blood-brain barrier while doing so.

The blood-brain barrier is a border that prevents pathogens from entering the central nervous system, or the brain. While hooked up to the heart-lung machine, this border had been down and a fungus from my old lungs had reached my brain and settled there.

"But there is some kind of medication for it, right? A pill I can swallow, right?" were the first questions I asked my neurology doctor. Since we finally knew what the problem was, now we only needed a cure for it: modern medicine.

"Well," my doctor said, and I immediately knew a simple pill wouldn't save me this time. "There is no pill for it. The problem is the blood-brain barrier. It also prevents medication from reaching the brain. The only medication we have available is IV. It's brand new from the US. We don't have any experience with it yet, but that's our only option. There is nothing else that could help. If this would have happened half a year ago, we wouldn't have been able to save you."

Suddenly I understood why my post-liver transplant doctor had been so rude to me when she told me I had to stay in the hospital right away. Half a year earlier, and I would have died. Because of a mushroom farm inside my head. I would have gotten more and more seizures. Not being able to flip a dice cup wouldn't have been my only problem. My personality would have changed, I would have lost connection to reality, and eventually I would have died.

There were not many jokes that afternoon while my mom and I sat in my room, waiting for my first anti-mushroom IV to be delivered that same day. It was a bitter pill to swallow (figuratively) to realize how many things could go wrong apart from the transplant itself. Getting new organs transplanted was almost the easiest part of it all. Getting the whole body back to working condition was a different story.

One of the nurses came in and hooked me up with my first anti-mushroom IV when I realized I finally got an answer to my ever-present question during my waiting time: Why did I have to wait that long for my transplant?

This was the reason. This IV was the reason. If I had been transplanted a few months earlier, maybe even after the three months the doctors had predicted as my waiting time, this IV would not have been available. If I had gotten the same fungus I had now, I would have died. Simple as that. Maybe God had known what he was doing and had kept an eye on me all that time. Maybe.

The IV was done within thirty minutes, and my mom and I went back downstairs to sit in the shopping street. I was ready to eat my obligatory Hawaii toast without Hawaii, and my mom was ready for more caffeine.

"I wonder if you can get a golden membership card for the café," she said on our way down.

"You mean like a loyalty card? You eat ten Hawaii toasts without Hawaii, and the eleventh is free?"

"Something like that, yes." She nodded. "Who knows how long we will have to be here this time. It's starting to be expensive taking care of you."

The new plan was, I'd get IVs twice a day and, in a week, we would do another MRI to see if the fungus was shrinking or at least not growing anymore.

"Maybe I'll get my own item on the café's menu," I said, our humor slowly coming back. "Like 'Inka toast.' Hawaii without Hawaii. And then I can eat as many as I want for free. Because it's my very own Inka toast."

"Yeah." My mom nodded again and held the door open for me. "With your luck, you'll get the mushroom soup named after you. Freshly grown all season."

Yes, it sucked. It all sucked. No one knew what to expect. No one even had an idea how long I'd have to get my anti-mushroom IVs. Weeks? Months? Years? But we were determined to make the most of it and sprinkle everything with a good dose of black humor. Especially the things that weren't funny at all.

The following days at the hospital could be summarized in one word: boredom. Besides my IVs in the morning and evening and my once-a-day physiotherapy, there was nothing to do but wait, until one afternoon, we met an old friend: Kat and her mom.

I had met Kat for the first time years back at a book presentation for cystic fibrosis. Back then we had talked a bit, both of us being diagnosed with CF, both of us living life to its fullest, both of us young teenagers. But even though we had a similar mindset on how to deal with a chronic disease, we had lost contact. And now here she was, at the shopping street of Hannover, walking around with her mom and killing time. Same as us.

"What a lucky coincidence," Kat's mom said when we ran into them, and we all felt the same. Finally, all of us had someone else to talk to beside our mom and daughter.

Kat's mom looked as she had all these years ago when we met her for the first time. Short, brown hair, taller than me but shorter than my mom, jeans, T-shirt, and the same ready-to-roll-up-your-sleeves attitude as my mom.

Kat, on the other hand, looked very fragile. She had always been short (half a head shorter than my 5"6' frame) but a powerhouse through and through. Now, all her strength was gone. She sat in a wheelchair, was much skinnier than I remembered her; hunched shoulders, shallow breath, composed movements not to burn too much energy, like a shell of what she had once been. Only her brown hair was short as always.

My mom and Kat's mom hit it right off. Getting another cup of coffee, settling into one of the few sofas beside the shopping street, while Kat and I did the same, only a few rows away from them. Our moms shared how hard it was to accompany dying children, and Kat and I talked about how hard it was to simply not die.

"I can't believe you're already transplanted," Kat said with a cough and a hint of jealousy. "I'm still waiting. Ugh, and it's so damn hard *and* boring."

"You're waiting here, in the hospital, high urgency?"

"Yes." She threw her arms up weakly. "Though I hope for not much longer. It's getting harder every day. You know what I mean."

I did. I looked at her wheelchair.

As a response, Kat patted the armrest of her contraption. "I only walk around when I'm upstairs in my room," she explained. "Breathing has become my enemy. At night, I even use a BiPAP to keep me going. It's been hard. Really damn hard."

I nodded because I didn't know what else to do or say. Kat was indeed in bad shape if she needed a BiPAP. It's a non-invasive ventilation. A mask is placed over the patient's mouth and nose, and the BiPAP uses positive pressure to help the patient breathe. It basically presses air into the patient's lungs because the patient can't breathe sufficiently any longer.

I had never used a BiPAP. I had never been that sick. I had never been as sick as Kat was.

I suddenly remembered my fellow CF patients from my second rehab in Amrum and how they had looked at me as if they all knew I wouldn't make it because I was that sick. Was I looking at Kat now with the same hopeless expression on my face?

I shook my head. No. Kat might have been sicker than I had ever been, but if someone could fight their way through, it was Kat. There was no doubt in my mind that she would make it. Probably even better, faster, stronger than I had. She just had to.

When we all went back to our floors, my mom and I were excited for the first time in what felt like years. It was great talking to someone else besides each other. It felt so good to talk to someone going through the same shit we had gone through. Finally, we had something to look forward to. Hawaii toast *and* nice company.

When my mom left to drive back to my aunt, I sat down and wrote another letter to Ingo. A good one this time:

> Dear Ingo,
>
> I'm slowly starting to feel my new life. I met an old friend today who's still waiting for her transplant, and for the first time, I realized how healthy I am. Compared to her I could see how my life is completely different now. It truly is. Suddenly I realize how I'm walking through the hospital all day without coughing, how I'm not tired anymore all the time, how I have a whole new life in front of me. (And no headaches.)
>
> Is this truly the beginning of my second life, my second chance? I'm almost afraid to ask out loud. It's not easy to accept the gift of a new life. Weird, right? When I still had to fight for my life, everything afterward seemed so clear, so easy. I knew what my new life should look like. What I would do with it. I knew everything. But now, since I don't have to fight for it anymore, I suddenly feel like I don't know anything anymore.
>
> Still, apart from all my doubts and worries, today was the first time I was able to feel my new life. To be able to feel myself again. To feel Inka again. I'm finding my

> direction, slowly getting reconnected to earth. Slowly arriving. Hurray!
>
> Still, I hope you will be with me for a little longer. To have a new life in front of you can be scary, as scary as fighting death. Sometimes even more. — Your not-yet-but-at-least-a-bit-reconnected-to-life niece

Despite our newfound company, days passed by as if carried by sleeping snails. We walked every existing hall inside the Medical School of Hannover. My mom could be a tour guide there if she ever felt the need to. We drank gallons of coffee, alone and together, and even with Kat and her mom. They were still waiting for her transplant, while I was still waiting to hear back if the anti-mushroom IVs were helping so I could go home.

My first MRI since I had started with the IVs had shown that my mushroom had stopped growing. Now we had to wait for the next MRI. If that one showed the mushroom was shrinking, I would be sent home with my IVs. I couldn't wait. Neither could my mom. But even though our minds were already on our way back home, I still went to physiotherapy every morning. After breakfast, after my IV was through, I went downstairs to the hospital's gym. Although *gym* was maybe not the right word for it. The gym consisted of one stationary bicycle, one treadmill, a few balls, a few weights, and a moderately enthusiastic physiotherapist who told me each morning what I had to do.

I normally spent some time cycling, then I walked for ten minutes on the treadmill, followed by throwing balls forth and back or lifting a few weights. It was nothing compared to the physiotherapy I got at my parents' place, but I moved my body and had something to do every morning.

While I spent my hours with the physiotherapist, my mom spent her time in the hospital's garden. On one of the first warm days of the year, everyone seemed to use the opportunity to spend some time outdoors. My mom walked around a little, down the paths she had already walked countless times, alongside neatly cut lawns, trees, and colorful flowerpots, until she found a bench that still was partly vacant.

"Can I sit?" she asked the young woman who was already sitting there. She had seen her a few times in the shopping street. As skinny as me, long, curly hair, askew glasses on her nose, hunched shoulders, seeming comfortable in a hospital setting. For sure CF as well.

"Sure," she said, then added: "You're Inka's mom, right? The one who had had a lung and liver transplant last year?"

My mom looked a little surprised but nodded. "Yeah, that's correct. You know her?"

"No," the young woman said, pushing her glasses up her nose again, "but I've heard of her. I'm also waiting for a lung transplant. Also CF. Do you mind if I ask you a few questions about how Inka's transplant went?"

Of course, my mom didn't mind. First, she was always ready to help others, and second, she was as desperate as all of us for anything that would make time pass faster than usual.

While my mom and the young CF patient were talking, another woman sat beside them. She was pushing a stroller with her one-year-old baby girl inside of it. It was obvious that the girl was the patient. She still had a feeding tube sticking out of her nose and looked fragile.

My mom smiled at the mom, remembering how I had looked right after my birth—also a feeding tube sticking out of my nose, and just as fragile.

"Yes," she said, turning back to face the CF patient, catching up where she had left off, "it's been almost four months since the transplant. It was on December twenty-eight. Early in the morning."

"Wow," the young woman said. "Already four months, and she looks so healthy. Thinking she got lungs and liver, that's just crazy."

The mom sitting beside my mom turned around, leaned closer, and raised her arm.

"Excuse me," she said. "I didn't mean to eavesdrop, but I couldn't help but hear the date. December twenty-eight. And the organs were lungs and liver?"

"Yeah . . ." my mom said, a little hesitant. "That's right. My daughter got lungs and liver transplanted on that day, last year."

"My daughter got a new liver on that day too," the woman said and scooched closer with a wide grin on her face. "Her surgeon told me it was a split liver. He also told me that the bigger part of her liver"—she pointed at her daughter—"including the lungs, went to a young woman that same day. That must have been your daughter."

There was silence for a moment. The young CF patient was speechless, same as my mom.

"So that means," my mom said, trying to catch up, "that my daughter and your daughter got part of the same liver?"

"Yes." The woman laughed out loud. "My name is Michelle, and this is Maya."

When I came back from physiotherapy, I found my mom still sitting outside on that bench and was immediately introduced to my liver-sister, Maya.

When the doctors in Hannover got the call for donor organs, they didn't know the liver they'd receive would be in such good shape that it could be split. But when they saw the liver, they immediately decided on it. Maya had only days to live. The chance they would find a pediatric donor in time to save her life was close to zero. Splitting the liver at hand was her only and last chance for survival, and it worked. My donor had not only saved two adults, but he had also saved a one-year-old baby girl. What a miracle.

We exchanged numbers and promised to stay in touch, which we did.

21

Punctured

One afternoon, the lung transplant doctors invited everyone post-transplant to a small gathering. To exchange stories, to get to know each other, and to support each other in finding our way back to life. I immediately liked the idea and joined.

We met in one of the meeting rooms normally reserved for doctors and professors and sat around a huge wooden table. There were seven transplant recipients, one of our many doctors, and two nurses.

It was nice hearing everyone else's transplant stories. Some told a story of easy transplants, quick recoveries; some had been even harder than mine. One of them had received a second lung transplant already. She had been in a coma for weeks before the transplant and was so weak afterward, she wasn't even able to lift an arm. But here she was, telling her story of resilience and the will to live. It was inspiring, and I was very happy I had come, until we reached the topic of how all of us had accepted our new organs.

One after another told their story of how they already felt like the new organ was theirs. That the new lungs felt like their lungs. Every such statement was accompanied by a content nod of doctor and nurses.

"It's very healthy to accept your new organ as your own," the doctor said. "This is where we want you to get. To the point of feeling whole again, that the new organ is yours."

"This is a very important step." One of the nurses chimed in. "You need to be able to trust the new organ. To trust that it won't stop breathing just because it was transplanted. To accept it as your own is a huge part of that trust."

Collective nodding, and then it was my turn to express how I felt about my new organs. Suddenly I wasn't so sure I liked the idea of sharing stories anymore.

"I don't see my new organs as mine," I said, hesitant at first, but growing stronger with each word. "I see my organs more like a rental. Something I can use for as long as I need to, but when I die, I will give them back because they aren't mine. I only use them; I don't own them. That's at least how I see it."

If I still had any doubt I wasn't Inka anymore, now I knew I was back to who I had been before the transplant. Always ready to swim against the stream. Always ready to steer the pot with an unorthodox opinion.

What followed was silence. No one said anything. No one commented on what I had said. We just continued the round with the next patient telling how they had already accepted their new lungs as their own.

Toward the end of our meeting, one of the patients was asked how he had gotten himself in a cast. His leg was fixated all the way up to his femur. Something you didn't see every day on a lung transplant recipient.

"I broke it while skiing," he said, followed by a collective, astonished gasp. Nobody could believe he had done something as dangerous and outrageous as skiing *after* a lung transplant.

"How reckless."

"Irresponsible."

"Way too dangerous for transplant recipients."

"I'd never do anything like that" were only some of the comments I heard, phrased by the nurses and patients.

I couldn't believe it either. Not because it was dangerous, but because I hadn't even thought of anything like skiing yet. Here I was, thinking of myself as oh-so advanced by not seeing the donated organs as my own, and hadn't even realized skiing was possible in the new life I got. As of now, all I had wanted for my new life was going back to university, moving into my own apartment again, and getting my dog back. But there was so much more out there. I finally had a new life; didn't I owe it to my donor to make the most of it?

"It is dangerous for transplant recipients to break a bone or get otherwise seriously injured," the doctors said. "Your immune system is compromised, your healing ability decreased, the risk for infections much higher than for any healthy person . . . it's just not worth risking a broken bone for a day on the slopes."

We all nodded, even though me and the guy with the broken bone knew our doctor was incorrect. A broken bone was definitely worth a day on the slopes. Because this was the reason all of us had gone through an organ transplant. To get a life. To live a life. And not only by sitting on a sofa, being safe. No, by living it to the fullest. Potentially broken bones included.

When I came back to my room after the meeting, my mom asked: "And? How was the meeting? Learned anything?"

"Definitely," I said. I finally understood what kind of gift I had received: a life full of opportunities. Now I only had to gather the guts to live it. To gather the guts to ski down that hill.

The next MRI showed that my fungus was indeed shrinking. The IVs helped, and I was scheduled to finally go back home. Only one procedure still had to be done: the placement of a port.

A port is a small medical appliance that's installed beneath the skin, normally right under the collarbone. A catheter connects the port to a vein, through which my IVs could be administered easily at home. Every three days, the membrane of the port, placed directly under the skin, would be penetrated with a needle from the outside. The needle would get fixed with a special Band-Aid to my shoulder and be used to connect the IVs. Until the needle had to be replaced again.

It was the perfect solution for a home IV therapy that could last for months or even years. No one knew how long I'd have to take these IVs; therefore, a port that could last for years was the perfect solution. No need to drive to a hospital in the middle of a Saturday night to get a new venous access. No need to worry about anything. Only problem: the port had to be placed first, under local anesthesia, and the surgeon who did it was nothing but a butcher.

Everything went wrong right from the start. The operating room I was supposed to be in was occupied. Instead, the surgeon decided to use the ER operating room. One nurse told him the ER operating room was equipped differently, that the right tools for placing a port were probably not available, but that was not a problem for my glorious surgeon.

"We'll bring everything we need from the other operating room over here," he told everyone, and unfortunately to me, no one had the guts to disagree with him.

Quickly everything needed was gathered, and I was placed on the operating table. The area around my collarbone was tapped off and sterilized, and my surgeon started to inject me with local anesthesia.

In the beginning, he was nice. Used all kinds of psychological tricks to keep my mind occupied and me distracted from what was about to happen. He asked me if I had a favorite book. What my hobbies were, if I was studying anything at university, things like that. But when the local anesthesia didn't work as fast as he had expected, he got nasty.

"If the shoulder isn't numb soon, there won't be much I can do but operate. Pain or no pain."

No one said anything. Not me, no nurse, no one. Also, my surgeon didn't ask me any questions anymore. Instead, he started to operate, and I started to pray my shoulder would stay numb and I would get out of there as soon as possible.

The atmosphere around me changed to busy attention. Everyone knew what they had to do; the train was back on track. I tried to occupy myself with counting. I couldn't see anything; the wrapping that covered my shoulder also covered my face, which made it hard to keep myself distracted.

"I will now insert the catheter into the jugular vein," the surgeon said, and I felt a tiny relief. We were almost done. The catheter had to be placed inside the vein, the port had to be fixed to my muscle, and I had to be stitched up. That was it. Almost done. Almost there.

If we had been in the right operating room and my surgeon had the right instruments. The right instruments that fit the size of my tiny veins.

But he didn't.

"This is never going to work," was the first thing he said. "This shit is way too small. I need way smaller instruments. I'll never get the catheter in like this."

Again, utter silence followed his words. I considered for a moment to just get up, show him the finger, and walk out of the operating room. But unfortunately, I wasn't bold enough to do any of that with a cut-open shoulder.

Before my surgeon could find additional suitable words for the situation at hand, the phone inside the operating room rang.

One of the nurses listened to what was said on the other end, and then she turned to my surgeon. "They want to know when the room will be free again. How long it will still take us to place the port."

"I don't know when I'll be done here," my surgeon barked back at her. "The way it looks, this will take forever."

A few minutes later, a second surgeon joined us. Maybe one of the nurses had called him to help, I didn't know. But together they came up with a genius solution: to puncture one of the bigger blood vessels and get the catheter in that way.

I just said, "Okay." I had been informed about this possibility beforehand and hoped surgeon number two was more capable than surgeon number one, when suddenly an unexpected bleeding occurred. Strong pressure was applied to my shoulder, and I was assured: "Nothing to worry about. Just a minor bleeding. We just have to stop it. Will only take a second."

By then, I started to concentrate on my breathing. I could feel how my body was getting ready to panic and did everything I could to stop it. I couldn't panic now. I had to stay calm. My panicking wouldn't help anything.

The bleeding stopped after about a minute of pressure, and then I felt it. A bubbling in the back of my throat. A bubbling I knew very well from my time before transplant. A bubbling that only meant one thing: lung bleeding.

The idiots had punctured my lungs. My new, transplanted lungs.

I immediately told the surgeons that my lung was bleeding, and they absolutely denied it.

"No, everything is okay. The lungs are okay. Nothing to worry about. We are almost done."

I wanted to scream at them. I wanted to slap them, wipe their arrogant behavior off their faces, and have them kicked out of the operating room. I wanted to bring in a surgeon who actually knew how to operate. But my body didn't let me.

Panic took over.

I started to sweat out of every pore. I was afraid I might pass out and, at the same time, tried to suppress any tears that were ready to wash me away.

The worst thing of it all was, I didn't have to panic. If the doctors had just told me the truth! Of course they had punctured my lungs, but it wasn't a big deal, I would have been fine. I wouldn't worry about my lungs being damaged. I wouldn't worry about being the victim of a disastrous medical mistake. I would have been calm.

But I was kept in the dark. The port was finally placed, and the surgeons congratulated themselves for being fucking geniuses. Only thing left to do: take an X-ray to assure that the catheter was in place. But even an X-ray was not possible without drama.

I still had the cover over my face, still couldn't see any of what was going on around me, while I was moved in the right position for my X-ray. I heard a buzzing noise, probably the arm of the X-ray machine being placed over my shoulder; the nurses around me were talking, moving around, being busy with whatever, when I saw something was pressing down the cover over my face, coming toward me, about to collide with my face.

That was when I screamed.

It was probably the arm of the X-ray machine still hovering above my face, and my coming toward it because the table I was lying on was moved upward. But I didn't know.

Whatever was on a collision course with my face was moved out of the way. The X-ray was taken, and I was stitched up, followed by the surgeon ripping off the cover from my chest and face and almost taking my nipples with it.

My mom was beyond happy when I rolled out of the operating room. Sure, I was as pale as a sheet of paper, but I was alive. The port placement should have taken thirty minutes. I had been inside the operating room for almost two hours.

When I was back in my room, I cried uncontrollably.

On March 24, I was finally released and on my way back home. I learned how to use my port, my mom had organized a fridge full of anti-mushroom IVs that were already waiting for me at their house, and life was falling back into place. I still had to go back to Hannover every week, later every two weeks, to get an MRI of my head taken, as my doctors were still nervous about that mushroom farm in my head.

But for the first time since my transplant, life seemed to calm down.

During this time, Kat finally got her new lungs. When we were back in Hannover a few days later, we immediately met with her mom to hear all about the good news. Kat's transplant went very well. After one day, the doctors had already taken her off ventilation and she was breathing on her own and responding to her surroundings. Everything looked perfect. She'd be back on her feet in no time. Way faster than I recovered. I knew it.

But when we were back in Hannover two weeks later, nothing was perfect anymore. Kat's health had declined more and more over the last two weeks to a point where her doctors had run out of options. The only comfort Kat's mom got was that Kat was not aware of what was happening. She was back on ventilation and sedated.

In the night, Kat's parents, together with my mom, went to see Kat for the last time and then turned off her life support. She lay in the same room I had lain in after my transplant.

Kat kept breathing for a few minutes before she passed.

In silence, Kat's parents and my mom went down and sat alongside the empty shopping street. But there was nothing to say, and nothing to do anymore. Kat's parents would drive home the next day, without their daughter. How? No one knew.

In May, my sister stopped by for a visit and brought my dog Fenja back with her. She had decided it was time for me to not only take care of myself, but also to take care of Fenja.

I was worried. Very worried. My muscles were still weak, and every evening I still felt drained from the day, but taking care of my dog helped a lot, much to my surprise. Fenja kept me moving. If the weather was bad, I still had to take her on a walk. If I felt tired, lazy, or unmotivated, the dog still needed to go outside. A huge portion of my recovery was due to her, my four-legged companion, but unfortunately, I couldn't tell Hannover about it. Not a single word.

Hannover was known for running a tight ship when it came to their organ transplant recipients. Every transplant recipient was indoctrinated to stay away from dirt, fur, fungi, and potentially dangerous activities. No skiing, no pets, no digging around in the garden, and oh dear God, no horseback riding. Horses were the equivalent to dust finding its way into airways, thus bringing death and gore. If it was up to Hannover, a perfect organ transplant recipient would stay home on the sofa, safe from life and live forever. Thank God I had never been a perfect patient.

Shortly after I got Fenja back, I picked up horseback riding again. I didn't do it for long, since riding had never been my thing, but since I was finally physically capable of riding, I was determined to give it a try. If we had had a mountain nearby, I might have also started skiing. I didn't allow myself to fear life just because I was an organ transplant recipient. And I didn't allow myself to believe in the fear my doctors preached:

"There can be fungus in garden soil—better not touch it."

"Dogs are dirty, carry bacteria around, and are potentially infested with worms and other parasites. Stay away."

"A broken bone might not heal after a transplant. Life-threatening complications can occur."

Fear was the main source of every rule I ever heard from my transplant doctors. As if the patient's cooperation couldn't be reached without it.

And I hated it.

I didn't want to be ruled by fear. I wanted to be ruled by knowledge and common sense. I had a brain—sure, it was infested with mushrooms—but still, I had a brain, *verdammt*, and I was determined to use it.

22

Gratitude

Every hospital all over the world followed the same routine when it came to checkup visits after transplant. But only Hannover managed to make every one of those visits as unpleasant as possible. Each visit started with first having my blood drawn. Followed by a pulmonary function test, oxygen saturation, an x-ray of the lungs, and last, waiting to see one of the doctors to be cleared to go back home. Only once I was cleared to go back home, I was allowed to eat. Every patient had to fast until cleared by the doctor because only the doctor could decide if a bronchoscopy was needed, or not.

During a bronchoscopy the doctor looked inside the lungs by inserting a tube through one's nose. This procedure was done every time the lung function wasn't perfect because a declined lung function could mean rejection. Any rejection had to be treated immediately to prevent lung damage and could only be diagnosed by bronchoscopy. And for a bronchoscopy one had to fast.

In 2003 it was still common practice to measure the oxygen saturation by blood. A blood circulation stimulating cream was applied to my ear, I had to wait five minutes, got poked, and the saturation was taken. It was always the same nurse who did this test, and she was always in the same, pleasant mood.

"No eating! No talking!" she barked at my mom and me after the cream was applied. "Any eating or talking will mess up the result."

She shot both of us a stern look, and was out the door, ready to return in five minutes.

"No eating, no talking, no breathing," I whispered at my mom and we both giggled.

"Be quiet," she said, shushing me. "I don't want to get in trouble."

"You think I'm allowed to dance? She didn't say anything about not dancing."

Five minutes passed, my blood was taken, and my oxygen saturation was perfect.

In the following years I would become a transplant patient of hospitals in Vienna, Austria. St. Louis, Missouri. Dallas, Texas and Denver, Colorado. Nobody ever cared if I talked, ate, danced, or sang an aria during my oxygen saturation test. Only Hannover.

Next, we went downstairs to get the x-ray taken. Also here, the same radiologist assistant greeted me with the same question every time: "Did you get small or big lungs?"

The radiologist assistant wanted to know how big the x-ray picture had to be.

And every time I answered: "I don't know. I was asleep when they put them in."

But radiology assistants don't have a sense of humor. I'd never find out if I had gotten small or big lungs.

My lung function test was next, and it showed that my lung function was still climbing. So far, I was at an FEV1 of 2.36 liters. An equivalent of about 70% of lung function. Pretty good.

Last, we saw one of the many lung transplant doctors and here, routine took over too. It was always the same questions I was asked:

"Did you have any infections or a cold since we last saw you?"

"Are you active during the day?"

"Do you eat enough?"

And my favorite: "How many stairs can you climb?"

I didn't know how many stairs I could climb. I never climbed stairs until I couldn't anymore. I was able to walk three miles with my dog, I was able to ride a horse for more than thirty minutes, all of it without being out of breath, but none of that I could tell my doctors.

"About a hundred?" I always said, asked, not sure how many stairs were enough, not sure how many stairs were many.

In 2018, I found the answer to that question by spending forty-five minutes in a gym on a stair master: "Two thousand seven hundred seventy-five stairs." But I'm sure in 2003 the number of a hundred was about correct.

I was released by the doctor without the need for a bronchoscopy and the request to come back in a month. From weekly checkups I had made it to monthly checkups. I truly was getting back to health day by day and with health coming back, also my confidence in me and my body returned.

Right after my transplant I didn't really know how to interpret any symptoms my body exposed. Before my transplant I always knew what was going on, if it was serious or could be ignored; after transplant everything was so new, everyone was always on edge, everything seemed serious. Any tiny hiccup was reason for concern, but as weeks passed by, as I got stronger and stronger, I developed a sense for my body again. I knew when it was okay for me to be out of breath. I knew when I needed rest and when I had to push myself a little further. I trusted life again, I trusted myself again, and, because of it, started to question my doctors. Just like I had before my transplant.

The first matter I took back into my own hands was the fasting during my checkup visits in Hannover. I knew my lungs were fine.

My home pulmonary function tests were always stable, there was no need for a bronchoscopy. Therefore, I ate, every time we went for a checkup, right after my blood work was done. Me and my mom sat down in the empty shopping street early in the morning, unwrapped our sandwiches we had prepared at my aunt's place, and dug in. We never got caught, until one morning.

We just sat down, my mom was still unwrapping her sandwich, I already took a huge bite out of mine, when my main post-transplant doctor walked past us. He was on his way to work. He still had his coat on, carried a briefcase, deep in thought, only sixteen feet away from us.

We both froze. My mom mid-unwrapping, I mid-chewing, hoping he wouldn't see us and just walk by. If he'd see us, I knew we would be in huge trouble. Nobody likes when their rules are literally chewed up and swallowed, especially no God in white.

He was almost past us, we were about to exhale, when he stopped in his tracks. Right there, right in front of us. I could see his forehead wrinkle; I could see how his glasses were still fogged up halfway as he looked back where he had come from. Like he had forgotten something. Maybe his lunchbox in his car.

I could hear my mom taking suppressed breaths beside me and prayed she wouldn't look at me. One glance from my mom and I would have burst laughing. Then my doctor would see us, burst into anger, maybe even refuse to treat me any longer as his patient. Who knew what he would do.

I saw his forehead unwrinkled again, for one more second he glanced into the distance, deep in thought, and then he finally kept on walking. Past us and around the corner.

The second he was out of sight, we laughed so much, I almost choked on my sandwich. It was the most fun we ever had in Hannover.

Every following appointment we sat further down the shopping street, always laughing thinking of the day we were almost caught eating sandwiches.

No bronchoscopy was done that day, as I had expected, and I would never get one done during my first year of post-transplant checkups because my new organs were doing great. Only one doctor thought differently.

It was a visit I did together with my sister. We followed the same routine my mom and I always did. Blood work, secret breakfast at the end of the shopping street, pulmonary function test, X-ray, and then going upstairs to see the doctor.

All my tests came back perfect. There was no indication for a bronchoscopy, or at least that's what I thought.

"I guess no bronchoscopy today," I told my doctor when we were almost done with our visit. I was all cheery because I had just passed another post-transplant checkup with flying colors, but my doctor only wrinkled her brows.

"We will see if we need to do a bronchoscopy or not," she said, still flipping through my test results.

"But why would she need a bronchoscopy?" my sister chimed in. "Don't the test results look great? As expected?"

"I don't want a bronchoscopy if there's no reason for it," I added, thinking of the two huge sandwiches I had eaten only two hours ago, which would become a problem if they truly wanted to take a look inside my lungs.

"If there's a bronchoscopy or not"—my doctor stood up—"is still my decision, not yours. I will be right back to tell you how we'll proceed."

The door closed behind her, and my sister and I exchanged confused looks.

"That poor woman seems to be confused." My sister said what I was thinking. "*If* there's going to be a bronchoscopy or not is *your* decision and *yours* only. *She*, on the other hand, doesn't decide anything."

"You think I can say no if they say they want to do one?" I was okay defying rules when no one saw it, but to confront one of my transplant doctors head on was a different subject altogether.

"Of course you can say no," my sister said with a sharp thrust of her chin. "And you should. There is no reason for them to look into your lungs. Unless they can explain to you why it's needed despite a perfect lung function test."

When my doctor came back, she told us she had decided a bronchoscopy wasn't needed after all and that I was allowed to drive back home. We left her believing *she* had decided. Doctors' egos are fragile—no need to mess with them.

When we were back in the car, my sister said, "Thank God I didn't have to make you puke out your sandwich for an unnecessary bronchoscopy. That would have been awkward."

Indeed, it would have been awkward. I was ready to take my health into my own hands again, but I was definitely not ready to explain to my doctors why I had to puke out a sandwich I wasn't allowed to eat to begin with.

When we got home, my mom had already received a call from one of the nurses of Hannover to tell me how I had to adjust my immunosuppression medication.

Immunosuppressant medication is highly poisonous. If I took too much, I could experience kidney failure. If I took too little, I could have an organ rejection. It had to be balanced all the time, which was why the level of my immunosuppressant medication was measured constantly. Every week we would send a tube of my blood to Hannover to have them check it. A nurse would call back a few days later with the newly adjusted dose of medication. Unless we had a checkup appointment. Then Hannover drew the blood themselves.

"What did they say?" I asked my mom, getting out of the car. "Do I have to adjust my dosage again, or is it stable for once?"

"It was weird," my mom said, scratching the back of her neck. "It was a doctor who called, and he said your level is at one-oh-four, but you should double your dosage to get your levels up to two hundred."

"Up to two hundred? But I'm supposed to be at one hundred. I'm perfect. What are they talking about?"

We went inside, my mom made some coffee, and all of us sat down, ate some cookies, and tried to figure out why that doctor had said such nonsense. Eventually, it was my dad who had the right idea.

"I know what happened," he said in between sips of coffee. We all looked up. "The level for the immunosuppressant is supposed to be at two hundred right after transplant, correct?"

We all nodded in agreement.

"Yours is supposed to be hundred because of the fungus in your head. To give your immune system a chance to help fight it besides the IVs, yes?"

More nodding.

"The doctor who called doesn't know you. He only saw the number one hundred, saw you were transplanted less than a year ago, and without checking your file, he assumed you needed to be at two hundred. Like everyone else. Simple as that."

From that moment on, we also took the adjustment of my immunosuppressant medication into our own hands. My mom, after calling everyone who had a phone inside the Hannover Medical School, found out the direct phone number for the lab doing the testing. We would call them every week to get my numbers and then decide over dinner how to adjust my medications.

When Hannover called to tell me how to adjust my medication, I just played along and said yes to everything they suggested. When I had a checkup appointment and the dosage they had written down versus what our family had decided on over dinner didn't match, Hannover always assumed an error in their notes.

They knew as well as everyone that the quality of their aftercare post-transplant was far behind their prestigious transplant surgeries.

My days were still mostly empty, filled with walks with the dog, playing cards with my mom, enjoying the food my dad cooked every evening, physiotherapy, some horseback riding, and occasionally meeting friends. I was desperate to move back out, to go back to university, but at the same time I knew I still had to take it slow. I wanted to run around and be a super-busy student on her way to graduation, but I couldn't. Not yet.

But I was able to write a letter to my donor family. I felt it was time to say thank you.

In Germany, the donor family and the recipient must stay anonymous. They unfortunately are not allowed to meet each other. Ever. In order to say thank you, I had to write an anonymous letter, send it to Hannover, Hannover would forward it to the one person responsible for any correspondence between donor family and recipient, she'd read the letter, make it further anonymous if needed, *and then* forward it to the donor family.

It was a complicated and somewhat frustrating process. One of my biggest wishes was and still is to meet my donor family, but I was ready to give it a try. Maybe they'd write back? Maybe I'd hear something from them? Maybe. I addressed the letter "Dear Parents" since I didn't know anything about them.

> Dear Parents,
>
> First, I hope I don't invade your life with my possibly unwelcome letter. But I feel the need to write to you, because due to the tragic accident of your son, I got a new life. Because your son or you agreed to an organ donation, I can walk around without an oxygen tank and have a future again. I can't even say how grateful I am to you and your son for that decision. On the other hand, I also feel a little insecure because I have so much reason for joy due to his tragedy. Maybe it helps your grief to know that someone can live because of the accident? I am very aware that I'm only living due to a tragedy.
>
> I wanted to let you know, I will always treat the life I got from your son as something precious. Even though I didn't know him, I hope he likes how something living came from his death. I will make the most of his gift—I will make it count. Two other patients' lives were saved by your son. An older man and a one-year-old baby.

> I at least wanted to say hello. There's so much more I'd like to say, but I don't know how to express my gratitude for your donation and my sorrow for your grief. It's hard to grasp how close life and death can be, and sometimes even reverse roles.
>
> I hope you can gain some joy and strength from this letter.
>
> With incredibly grateful wishes, from a 24-year-old woman

I never received a letter from my donor family even though I wrote many more, but years later I met the person who took care of all the correspondence between recipients and donor families. She told me my donor family had always accepted my letters with joy but never felt ready to write anything back.

I was able to make peace with it. I still wished the rules in Germany were more like the ones in the US, where donor family and recipient can meet if they both agree to it, but the most important step I was able to take: share my gratitude.

23

Hospital . . . Again

When summer came around, I decided it was time for me to figure out how to pick up on studying again—this time in Düsseldorf instead of Oldenburg.

Oldenburg, where I went to university before, was about two hundred miles away from where my parents lived. Düsseldorf was only thirty miles away. I didn't feel comfortable to be two hundred miles away from my parents. I wanted to have them close, to know they could be with me in half an hour. That's why I chose Düsseldorf.

I sent a letter, asking the university of Düsseldorf to accept me as a psychology student in my fifth semester, and they said no. They didn't have space. The fifth semester was full for the upcoming fall and winter semesters. I would have to wait until summer semester next year and hope for a space then. But I didn't want to wait. I had waited enough. I had lost already two years because of my transplant. I didn't want to lose another.

I wrote a heartfelt letter in which I expressed my objection to accepting their decision and decided, instead of sending it via mail, to drive to Düsseldorf and deliver it in person. I was ready to give an emotional presentation of why I deserved a place at their university and wouldn't leave without it. But unfortunately, this wasn't a movie in which dreams come true. No, this was reality, and reality looked awfully bureaucratic.

The hall in front of the student guidance office where I headed to was crammed with other students. They were all waiting to talk to someone in that office, and they all looked as if they had already been waiting for some time.

I stood waiting in between all the other students in the hall, as they were to be the next in line, but I quickly felt overwhelmed. Standing so close to so many people made me worry I might catch a cold from someone. There were no chairs available to rest for a moment; some students sat on the carpeted floor, but I still felt too fragile. For sure there was a ton of dirt on that carpet, bacteria, maybe even fungus. No way I could wait here with all the others to get my turn to talk to a university representative and stay healthy. Maybe I wasn't ready for reality yet?

Defeated, I left the hall and went back to stand in the stairwell, when my eyes landed on the directory: Floor 1, room 90 — Dean of Psychology.

Without hesitation, I pressed the button for the elevator and rode upstairs to see the dean.

When the elevator doors opened, I was presented with a completely different view than the one from downstairs. I was greeted by an empty, freshly air-conditioned hall, nice couches on the right and left, shiny marbled floors, and a long line of shut, wooden doors.

I knocked on door number ninety and was called in. But it wasn't the dean himself who welcomed me—it was his secretary.

I wanted to bite my ass. I had not expected a secretary as a gatekeeper. But here she was. I first had to talk my way past her before I would be able to talk to the dean himself.

"Excuse me," I said. "I was sent up here from the downstairs office. I was denied a place in the fifth semester of psychology this upcoming fall, but I'm a special case and the ladies from downstairs sent me up here to talk to the dean himself."

A complete lie, but I didn't care. I *was* a special case. I deserved a place. And I would get a place.

The secretary took the letter I had prepared, read through it, agreed I was a special case, and then asked me who I had spoken to downstairs.

"Oh," I said, slowly exhaling, trying to buy some time to come up with the next lie. "I-I don't remember. It was a woman. This much I know."

"I'll call downstairs to verify," the secretary said, and I started to sweat.

Of course, the ladies downstairs had no idea who I was or who I had spoken to, but one of them wasn't in the office that day, so we all agreed that it must have been exactly that woman I had spoken to yesterday. I hoped she wouldn't get in trouble as I was sent through the next door to see the dean himself.

Like all the deans I had ever met, the dean of psychology in Düsseldorf was a man past his sixties, with thin gray hair, respectable clothes, a dark gray tie, horn-rimmed glasses, and a confused look on his face.

"Yes?" he asked, looking at his secretary for clarification on who I was and why I was entering his office.

"This young lady was denied a place in the fifth semester of psychology for the following quarter and wants to enter objection due to her being a special case."

"But . . ." The dean tried to enter objection himself, but his secretary had already closed the door behind me and returned to her desk.

His eyes landed on me.

"Please," he said, offering me one of the wide leather chairs in front of his desk. "Tell me what it is you need from me."

I summarized my story as quickly as I could, while the dean crossed his arms, leaned back in his even wider leather chair, and tapped the carpet under his desk. But the more I told him, the less he tapped and the more he leaned forward, until his elbow rested on his desk and his eyes were wide open.

"Dear God," he eventually said, "you truly have been through a lot. You'll make a good psychologist." He nodded, as if to reassure himself, then scribbled something on a blank piece of paper. "I'll get you in for the upcoming semester. I just have to find out how. You will receive a letter in the mail. It was nice talking to you. All the best, and *Gesundheit.*"

A week later, I got a letter in the mail. I was accepted as a new student of the Heinrich Heine University in Düsseldorf. My paper said I would start in the third semester because the fifth was truly full, but I could continue as planned where I had stopped in 2001. I was elated!

The following weeks, my dad and I drove to Düsseldorf almost every day and looked for an apartment for me. And eventually we found one.

It was a one-bedroom apartment with huge windows, a small balcony, and light fishbone parquet. Two supermarkets and a huge park lay a few hundred feet away; plus, my new home wasn't far from the university. It was perfect.

I moved in on a Wednesday. Surrounded by boxes, exhausted as hell, I felt like I was on top of the world. I had truly done it.

I was transplanted.

I was a student again.

I was living alone. (Together with my dog.) In a new city full of students I was ready to meet. I still had to take my twice-daily IVs for the mushroom farm inside my head, but I would manage. My plan was to start slowly. To only take a few courses in university, to get back into it, but otherwise to concentrate on getting to know people and getting used to an independent lifestyle again.

But before university started, I drove to visit Martina for a long weekend. I hadn't seen her in person since my transplant, and of course she couldn't wait to actually see and finally hug me. For the weekend, we had very specific plans: We wanted to do exactly what we had done before my transplant. Watching TV, eating cheese, talking about serious stuff and nonsense—only this time with a future to look forward to. We had so much fun and enjoyed every second, until I got a high fever on my second day.

After countless phone calls with my parents and doctors, Martina drove me to Hannover and the port was removed. It was infected. Somehow bacteria had found its way into it, and it couldn't be saved. My port was history.

I had to stay for a few nights in Hannover. My mom came to stay with me, as usual, and then my doctors decided it was time to discontinue my anti-mushroom IVs.

"You still have to come once a month for an MRI," one of the doctors told me. "To check that the fungus is not coming back, but other than that, we'll just keep our fingers crossed. No new port, no more IVs."

I wanted to jump off the roof, I was that happy. I had taken IVs for over half a year and now, right at the beginning of my new life, I got rid of them. It was the best thing that could've happened to me.

Two days after I had been released from the hospital, I had an appointment with my primary care physician (PCP) to check the scar from the port removal. After that appointment, I wanted to finally drive back to my apartment in Düsseldorf. So far, I had stayed with my parents to continue unpacking and getting ready for my first day at university that upcoming Monday. But when I arrived at the office of my PCP, he didn't even look at my scar. The scar was forgotten because suddenly I had excruciating stomach pain.

My PCP did an ultrasound and immediately knew what was going on.

"You have a bowl obstruction," he informed me. "We need to call Hannover. This"—he pointed at my belly—"needs to be operated today."

I was in too much pain to complain or whine about it. If he would've said he'd cut me open right then, I would've agreed. The pain was that bad. But instead, an ambulance was called, and I was transferred to the hospital where I had been with my stomach bug before transplant. My mom was already there waiting for me when I arrived.

"A bowel obstruction?" she said when she saw me, one eyebrow pulled up.

I only shrugged. What was there to say? I myself was still dizzy from the roller coaster I had been on for the last few days. Looking forward to being a student again, visiting Martina, high fever, port removal, no more IVs, and now a bowel obstruction, including operation ahead. I couldn't believe it either. I wanted to pull a joke, to lighten up the misery I had found myself in. Tell my mom to cheer up, get some popcorn, and enjoy the abdominal episode of *Fun at the ER with Inka*.

But I couldn't. Not even one miserable joke came to my mind.

All I wanted was painkillers, but painkillers slow down bowel movements. And I needed a bowel movement if I wanted to get rid of an obstruction. Therefore, I was left in pain and Hannover was called again.

After an X-ray and, thank God, a small dosage of painkillers, my PCP's diagnosis was confirmed: It was indeed a bowel obstruction, and Hannover wanted me transferred to their care.

"We will transfer you to Hannover immediately." The ER doctor came to my bed to inform me what Hannover had said. I wanted to remind them I had university this upcoming Monday, but my mom cut me off.

"Immediately?" she asked. "Does that mean they'll operate on her in Hannover the moment she arrives?"

"This . . ." The ER doctor shrugged. "I don't know. They should operate on her immediately, but that's up to them. By 'immediately,' I mean they will send a helicopter. You'll fly to Hannover."

"By helicopter?" Screw university, I couldn't believe my luck. "This is awesome."

"This is horrible," my mom said at almost the same time. "I don't want to fly in a helicopter. Not. At. All."

"What if they serve coffee and cookies?" I asked. After all, my mom was as food-driven as I was. But not this time.

"And if they serve salmon sandwiches and champagne, I don't want to fly."

"I don't think you'll have to worry about it," the ER doctor said. "What I heard, these helicopters don't have space for anyone besides the patient, the pilots, and a doctor. Not even salmon sandwiches."

And he was right. My mom couldn't fly with me; she had to drive to Hannover. No space. Also, no sandwiches.

We only waited for fifteen more minutes, and then were told the helicopter had landed. Right in front of the rural hospital. And because it didn't happen often that a helicopter landed at its front door, anyone who was still able to walk, crawl, or move had gathered to witness this exciting event. Patients, guests, nurses, even a few doctors.

When I was rolled outside to the helicopter pad, lying on a gurney, I saw many surprised and maybe even disappointed faces. I was sure everyone expected a traffic accident victim, unconscious, covered in bandages, tubes everywhere, leaving a trail of blood dripping from open wounds behind. Instead, they saw me, clearly in pain but otherwise unharmed, conscious, and laughing with the doctor who would accompany me to Hannover.

My gurney was secured inside the helicopter, and my mom quickly said her goodbyes to me.

"I'll see you in Hannover," she called after me, and I was sure if the doctor had offered her a seat inside the chopper, she would have jumped in without a moment of hesitation. Despite her fear and the disappointment of no salmon sandwiches, she would have come along just to be with me.

We both knew I would arrive in Hannover first. Which meant I could be lying on the operation table already when she arrived. An idea my mom sure wasn't fond of. She had always accompanied me till the last moment, and now I was sent ahead. From experience, we knew bowel obstruction surgery was a fairly big deal. As a newborn, I had survived my first one and still carried the scar from it, being now the length of almost ten inches, running vertical down my stomach. Having this kind of surgery now, not even one year after my transplant, was concerning to say the least. I hoped my mom would drive carefully but didn't have the chance to tell her. The doors of the helicopter closed, and while the engine warmed up, my doctor gave me another dosage of pain medication. At least in this regard, I was in heaven.

While we lifted off, I could already tell the pain medication had taken over, and soon after exhaustion did the same. I slept most of the flight and only woke up when we were approaching the landing pad of Hannover. Where I had seen many helicopters land throughout the last year and now would touch down myself. Sometimes it was hard to catch up with life.

When my mom finally made it to Hannover, she was surprised I wasn't cut open yet but placed in an ordinary hospital room.

"What's going on?" she asked when she rushed through the door, covered in sweat and in disarray but relieved to see me.

"The ER doctor heard a bowel movement." I smiled. "They hope it will clear itself without an operation."

"That's great!" My mom sat down beside my bed, finally relaxing.

After so much we had been through with doctors, we still believed shit when we heard it. Sad, but true.

When my mom came to see me the next morning, after she had spent yet another night at my aunt's house, nothing had changed. I was still in constant, excruciating pain and my doctor was still a big believer of having everything under control. I got enemas, I was rolled to get an X-ray multiple times to see if the contrast medium, a special kind of dye I swallowed earlier, was moving through my bowel, but it didn't. Nothing moved. Nothing. Every few hours I was allowed a pain medication IV that allowed me to sleep. Every time the last drop of the IV was through, I would wake up from pain again, suffering, not knowing where to put myself.

Eventually, it was already afternoon, and I said to my mom, "You gotta do something. Something has to happen. I'm so exhausted. I need to sleep. I can't be in this kind of pain for much longer."

And that was the moment it hit my mom. Something was going terribly wrong here, and she was the one who had to put it right because I was at the end of myself.

"I will take care of it." She stood up, left the room, and . . .

My mom didn't remember what she said when she left my room. She only remembers how everyone standing around—nurses, patients, my doctor—went completely silent and then things started to move. Very quickly.

My mom was barely back inside my room when the door opened again and the chief physician poked his head in. He didn't come in to examine me, didn't ask any questions—he only looked at my pain-stricken face and said: "Oh, shit." Literally.

Within minutes, my room was filled with doctors and nurses. A kidney transplant was pushed back, and at 9:01 p.m., I was back on the operating table. For a bowel obstruction. As my PCP had predicted already a day prior.

While I was cut open once again—literally because I was full of shit—my mom went to sit in the deserted shopping street and called my dad. She asked him to drive to my apartment in Düsseldorf, go through my unpacked boxes, and find my advanced healthcare directive. In it was written what kind of life support measures I agreed to and which I disapproved of. In case I would ever find myself unable to decide for myself.

My mom had a very bad feeling about the operation. She wanted to have my advanced healthcare directive handy in case she needed it. In case . . . I needed it.

My dad jumped into his car, drove to my still unpacked apartment in Düsseldorf, and got to work. Suppressing any thoughts about how I might never unpack the boxes he was going through right now. How my planned life in Düsseldorf might never start.

This was the hardest he ever had to do for me. The one that pained him the most.

While my dad was at my apartment, alone with the fear of losing his daughter once again, my mom called Tina.

"I need you here in Hannover," she told my sister. "I have a bad feeling about this. I need you. Right now."

And then my sister jumped into her car, met my dad on the way to pick up the advanced healthcare directive he had eventually found inside one of my many folders, and drove to Hannover.

Arriving in Hannover, my sister met my mom and they both stayed seated in the deserted shopping street. Only once in a while a doctor or a nurse walked by. Besides that, it was depressingly quiet.

"Here," my sister said. "Eat something." Tina handed our mom one of the sandwiches she had brought.

My mom did eat, even though she didn't want to, and just as she had finished her sandwich, her phone rang. It was my surgeon calling.

"Hello," he said, followed by, "Where are you right now?"

All the color drained from my mom's face. She looked at my sister, shook her head, and then asked: "She didn't make it?"

For a moment there was silence at the other end until the doctor realized how his question must have sounded to my mom.

"Oh, no, she is fine," he said quickly, apologizing and trying to set things straight. "She's almost back from surgery. Everything went well, but I wanted to talk to you in person if you could come up to floor five." If possible, even more color drained from my mom's face as she heard her biggest fear had not come true. I was still alive.

"We are on our way." My mom hung up, ready as usual to tackle the next step, but also feeling drained and weak. The last hours had taken their toll.

When my mom and sister reached floor five, they met the patient who was still waiting for her kidney transplant because of me. They exchanged a quick hello and a "good luck!" and then my mom slid once again down to the floor while leaning against the wall. Another nail to her coffin, she would later say.

The recovery from my bowel obstruction was both quick and difficult. Quick, because the bowel was fine and didn't get damaged. One day after, I was already standing beside my bed, shaking my naked butt to the music coming from the nurses station, which I don't remember. Thank God. Difficult, because my liver didn't agree with the huge operation I just had. My liver parameters were skyrocketing, nobody knew why, and fear spread that my liver got damaged in the process of saving my life.

An hour-long ultrasound was made, and multiple doctors were called to give their opinion, but eventually my liver, my doctors, and I calmed down. On November 7, I was allowed to go back home, but the incident of my bowel obstruction wasn't forgotten that quickly.

The doctor who had overlooked my bowel obstruction for a whole day had to answer some very uncomfortable questions during the following days, and everyone in Hannover knew about it. When my mom went to buy me another Inka toast during one of our following visits, the cashier asked her, "How is your daughter doing?"

My mom looked a little puzzled but answered her. "She's doing good. Just here for an MRI. Do you know her?"

"Oh." The cashier laughed. "Everyone knows *about* her and the bowel obstruction."

Yes, everyone had heard about me and how Hannover had almost let their first successful double lung and liver transplant recipient die because of a bowel obstruction.

Physically, I recovered very fast from my bowel obstruction and moved quickly into my apartment in Düsseldorf. My mind, however, was a different story.

24

A Seed

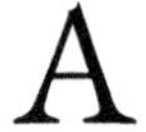

Another letter:

Dear Ingo,

It's been a few days since I've been back home, at my home, at my apartment in Düsseldorf. My stomach looks like ground beef after the last surgery. Cut open, from chest to pelvis bone, just when everything was finally healed. But what's worse, the inside of me looks the same. Chopped up. Cut to pieces. And then stapled back together.

I can't even describe how lost I feel. How can I ever trust my body again when I'm cut open and stitched back together all the time? When there's no security in life? Not even after transplant?

I hoped to lose my fear of death after transplant. Finally be able to catch up a little. But instead, I had to fight for my life again, from one day to another, without a warning. I didn't expect that. All the trust I had in my body is gone. I was sure I'd feel it if something were wrong, I was sure I would detect if something wasn't working, but I didn't. Instead, I'm afraid life could run through my fingers at any moment. Every little twitch in my stomach makes me doubt, instills fear to be cut open again. To see the operating lamp looming over me—again.

I don't want to be cut open again! I want my body to myself, healed. I don't want to see myself stapled together like a piece of meat. STOP THAT! I SUFFERED ENOUGH! LEAVE ME ALONE, ALL OF YOU!

But how do I reconnect with life? How can I find trust again if I only swing from life to death and back? How?

Maybe it's stupid to ask you this question, but I don't know who else to ask. I never felt as lifeless as now. It's as if God had personally sent me back to life but forgot to tell me what I'm supposed to do with it. All meaning is gone. Everything seems empty around me.

Sometimes I think maybe I should have just let go and died. Sometimes I don't even know why I fought so hard for another chance. For what? Do you remember? — Your feeling-empty niece

Beside my deceased uncle, there was only one other person I told about my struggle: Martina. We talked over the phone almost every day. She was my shoulder to cry on, and during one of these phone calls, she said something that made me think.

"You can't live with the consciousness of a sick person anymore; you need to start living like a healthy person."

When I heard these words for the first time, I wanted to scream. What stupid advice. *Live like a healthy person*—duh. Easier said than done. I had lived with a chronic disease for twenty-four years. I had always been *the* CF patient. I had popped pills, coughed my lungs out, been told I needed more rest than others; I had been to countless doctors' appointments, had needles plunged into me, and so many other things representing sickness. How could I go from that to believing I was healthy? Especially when popping pills and going to countless doctors' appointments still determined my life?

I still popped pills, I still had many doctors' appointments, and I still needed more rest than others, but deep inside of me, I knew Martina was right. I had to say goodbye to my sick life and start living the life of a healthy person. Popping pills had to become something I had to do, but not the thing that determined who I was in life. I didn't want to be the CF patient anymore, as little as I wanted to become the transplant recipient. Instead, I wanted to be healthy, to believe I was healthy, and to act healthy. I didn't want to use my disease as an excuse anymore for not being able to do things. I wanted to be burdened with all the things healthy people were burdened with because I was too. I wanted to build my life with a healthy mindset. With the belief that everything was possible while, of course, also being a responsible organ transplant recipient. But how? This was the question Martina didn't have an answer for either.

The first thing I did on my way to health was write in my diary again. Every day I wrote down what I had believed in, and what my thoughts had suggested for me to believe in. I tried to completely block out thoughts like, *I can't do this, I'm not strong enough, I'm a transplant recipient*, or *I'm weak and need to rest.* I only wanted to believe in me being strong, healthy, and resilient despite being a transplant recipient, but man, it was difficult. Fear and doubt were so much easier to conjure than belief and trust. But thank God, I might have lost my belief in myself after the bowel obstruction, but not my stubbornness. I was determined to get my brain rewired. Even if I had to fill a hundred diaries with entries like these:

> November 28, 2003
>
> So far, my thoughts are still torn apart. Not in harmony with my feelings. My subconsciousness still hangs on to my old life. I can feel it trying to rip me apart. Stuck between *I'm healthy and therefore resilient* and *I'm sick and therefore tired.* Maybe that's why I'm not ready to go back to university yet. I'm still recovering from my bowel obstruction and pushed everything one semester back. I'll start next semester. I first have to find myself again before I can concentrate on something else. Writing helps a lot, though. It feels as if for one moment I have found myself again. As if all the parts are reconnected for one moment. Once I put the pen down, they all fall back apart; but each time, one little piece stays in place. Slowly, I'm placed back together and start to trust myself again. Sloooowly . . .

> November 30, 2003
>
> It's not easy being healthy. It's easier being sick. I realize that every day. When you are sick, you always have an excuse. Always an explanation why you didn't try hard enough. Why you failed. Especially through my dreams I realize I'm not ready yet to be healthy. From time to time, I dream of Hannover. I dream of being sick again, lying on the operation table, gasping for breath. But I don't want to be sick anymore. I was sick long enough. I want to give my sickness back, but my head isn't ready yet. I'm writing I'm healthy, but my head is not convinced. It feels as if the seed to be healthy is planted, but it hasn't spread its roots yet to every corner of myself. The seed is still small and buried deep, and I have to check every day if it's still there. As long as I can feel that little seed, I know I'm on the right track.

For months and months, I filled diaries with words like these. Repetition was key. The more often I wrote I was healthy, the more often I was able to believe in it and feel it. And the more days, weeks, and months passed without my being admitted to a hospital, the further the roots of my healthy seed spread.

In 2004, I reached the point where I trusted my health enough to finally go back to university—exactly one semester later than originally planned—and finish my psychology degree. It felt good moving forward, being productive, and having to fulfill requirements again.

I tanked my first psychology test gloriously. For the longest time, nothing had been asked of me besides staying alive. There had been no task I had to fulfill besides that one. Now, I had papers to finish, tests to study for, homework assignments to turn in, and no disease to blame failure on. That ship had sailed. If I wanted to be healthy, I had to live my life without being presented with an extra cystic fibrosis or transplant recipient bratwurst. That's what we call special treatment in German: getting an extra bratwurst. It took me some time to say no to that extra brat, but eventually I got there, and it felt great.

The year 2004 ended without a single hospital stay. My FEV1 was at 3.12 liters, my liver parameters were normal, and Martina's idea turned into a new life motto: "You become what you believe you can become." And I started to believe I could become completely healthy one day. In my darkest hours, I hoped my newfound belief in my health and all the dreams that came with it wouldn't bite me in the ass later. It was good to believe in my health—I was rarely afraid of hospital visits anymore—but with all this came a certain amount of recklessness, which started to show in the beginning of 2005.

Believing in my health while paying attribute to being an organ transplant recipient made me walk a thin line between self-confidence and humility. I was ready to take control of my life again, especially regarding doctors' visits, but how much control was too much, and how much too little?

It was during one of my routine checkup appointments in Hannover, beginning of 2005. My mom and I were already sitting upstairs at the doctor's office, waiting for him to arrive to discuss my tests results, when he only poked his head in. "The chest X-ray is missing.

Before I can see you, you must go down and get your X-ray taken. Once you're back, I'll come see you."

He was about to close the door behind him when I said, "I know the chest X-ray is missing. I didn't get an X-ray today. I don't want to get an X-ray every three months. I'll skip every other. Next visit, I'll get one again."

My doctor stood still for a few seconds. Frozen in place and not able to believe what he had just heard. A patient telling *him* which tests were to be taken? That had definitely never happened before according to the look on his face.

I knew the risks that came with that decision. The X-rays weren't only taken to have a look at the lungs, they were also taken to be able to detect any form of cancerous growth early on. The immunosuppressant medicine I took, the one that made sure my body wouldn't reject my new organs, also presented a higher risk of getting cancer, so they routinely scheduled X-rays. But I didn't want that many X-rays taken for the rest of my life. Moreover, I was ready to take the risk of an undetected cancer growing in my lungs in exchange for fewer pictures. My doctor did not share this belief.

"I will not," he said with an angry tremor in his voice, "continue this conversation. Either you get an X-ray right now, or you can go home because I won't treat you any longer."

With that, he closed the door behind him and left me and my mom alone.

We looked at each other, dumbstruck, and then got up to follow him out the door.

He was still there, standing in the hall, trying to digest what had just happened, when my mom and I confronted him.

"I would like to at least discuss the number of X-rays . . ." I started a little shaky but determined to stand my ground. My doctor, however, was not ready to have *any* conversation about X-rays.

"If we would have known," my doctor said, his voice nearly a growl, "that you would cooperate that little after transplant, we would have not transplanted you."

I flinched and took a step backward, unable to believe what I had just heard. My mom and I stood speechless.

Before we could find our voices again and express the anger we both felt, another doctor, the one who had almost caught us eating sandwiches downstairs in the shopping street, came running and separated us.

I don't know if it was our body language that made him come over, or if the offensive words of the doctor who didn't want to discuss X-rays had traveled all the way to where he was standing. But my mom and I were ushered back into the examination room we had come from, and my doctor was sent to the next, hopefully more cooperative patient.

The doctor who had separated us took his place and promised me he would talk to the other transplant doctors to see if there was a possibility to lower my number of X-rays taken throughout the year.

That's all I wanted. To talk about it. Patients have rights too. The right to discuss treatment plans with the doctor, and the right to decide against the doctor's recommendation. Starting in 2006, I only had one X-ray of my lungs taken per year. Because it was *my* choice.

I was never treated by that doctor again who had said Hannover wouldn't have transplanted me if they had known how little I would cooperate afterward. Probably a good thing. Why argue with someone who believes he is God, when you believe he's close to nothing? But still, I would have loved to tell him a little bit about the amount of cooperation I had shown in my life.

I had been running almost my whole life to get the thick mucus out of my lungs that was slowly suffocating me. I even ran when the coughing was so bad that I had to throw up because of it. I ran even though I got nosebleeds from the coughing. I ran when I had a fever or was otherwise unwell. During my waiting time for my transplant, I went to the gym every day, even though I had barely enough energy to eat. I lived for fifteen months with the fear of dying at the age of twenty-three. I worked my ass off to get back on my feet, and then a doctor, whose worst disease had probably been the flu, had the audacity to tell me I wasn't cooperating enough? Sorry for my language, but: "Fuck you!"

In the summer of 2005, I threw a party for all my friends and family who had helped during the waiting time for my transplant and the time right after. We celebrated in my parents' garden with finger food, sitting on beer garden benches, music in the background, beautiful weather, and many stories to share and remember. It was a wonderful opportunity to say thanks to everyone and to express all the gratitude I felt toward my friends, my family, and my donor.

In the evening, when only the closest friends were left, my parents' garden was suddenly filled with fireflies. Green fireflies lighting up the lawn. It was the most bizarre and magical moment of that day. We rarely have fireflies in Germany.

The next day, I wrote my last letter to Ingo:

Dear Ingo,

Yesterday, I said thank you to everyone who had been with me during my waiting time. To everyone who had suffered and hoped with me. But one huge thank-you is still missing, the one for you:

I want to thank you for all the letters I wrote to you. For me being able to complain and whine to you and how you always held my hand, symbolically speaking. Your *presence* was the most wonderful present you could have given me. Thank you!

But unfortunately, my time of writing letters has ended. I miss you like never before. I never wished so much to have met you. At least hugged you one time. Seen you one time. In person, in real life.

But the time for letters has come to an end. I will say goodbye now. I won't write again.

But one thing I have to say before I leave: The seat beside you on cloud nine, it's mine. One day I will sit beside you and tell you all about the adventures that are still waiting for me. — Your moved-to-tears-and-forever-grateful niece

This is where my book was supposed to end. I survived my transplant. I established a new belief in my health and my abilities. I was on my way to becoming a psychologist. What else could there be to write about?

Well, as so often in life, everything got messed up when I met a man and he made me believe in a dream so big and so huge, I had never even thought of it.

25

Phone Book

It was a Friday, November 18, 2005, and I was out celebrating the birthday of one of my friends from university. We first met at her place, cooked some dinner, and then all of us got ready to go to a nearby club in the city of Düsseldorf, to the Les Halles.

The Les Halles was a really cool and unique club. Located on the outskirts of an industrial area, it presented itself as a mixture of a gothic living room, dancefloors, and French café, all of it cramped into an abandoned house. You could dance, sit on a sofa and observe, or sit in the French café at a small table and eat one of the few snacks the club offered.

The crowd was a wild mix too. Students danced beside Düsseldorf's high society, danced beside white-collar employees, danced beside white-collar foreign employees. And one of them decided to come over and talk to me.

"Hi," he said, or mostly screamed in my ear to be heard over the music around us. "My friend told me you speak English?"

He was not tall, about my height, jeans, a white button shirt, light stubble, and a confident grin on his face. *Cute,* I thought.

"A little," I answered truthfully. Everyone in Germany must learn English at school. There is no way around it. But I had never used my

English after school. I had never read an English book; I had never watched an English movie.

I was very rusty.

But the man in front of me didn't care. He just kept on talking. Telling me something about himself, his work, how much he liked the club. We danced a little bit, and his friends kept an eye on us. My friends paid even more attention, until he asked:

"Can I have your number to call you tomorrow?"

I hesitated. "My . . . number?"

I had had a few dates in the last months, and because of them, I was not really interested in meeting another member of the opposite sex. I was tired of excuses why someone hadn't shown up to a date, tired of hearing someone had *unfortunately* forgotten their wallet at home, and especially tired of exchanging texts that had no content whatsoever.

I was about to say no, about to blow him off, when I had an idea.

"I won't give you my number," I told him. "But I will give you my name. If it's important to you, you can find my number in the phone book. If not, not." The number of my landline, to be correct. No text messages whatsoever.

He looked at me a bit confused, obviously unsure if he understood correctly what I had said in broken English. But then nodded.

"Okay," he said. "I'll find your number and call you tomorrow. I have no idea how a German phone book works, but I'll figure it out."

That's exactly what I had been aiming for. He had to give effort in order to take me out on a date. If I was worth the effort.

One of my friends ran off to get me a pen and a small piece of paper where I scribbled my name on. *Inka Rasch.* He was lucky my name wasn't the German equivalent of Mary Smith. There was only one Inka Rasch in all Düsseldorf.

He took the note with a decisive nod, wrote his name at the bottom, and ripped the lower part off for me to take home: Eli Nisinbaum. For sure the only one in all Düsseldorf and foreign indeed.

It was Saturday afternoon, and I was chilling on my sofa, not thinking of anything, especially not about Eli of last night, when my landline rang.

"Rasch," I answered.

There was a short moment of silence, then: "Hi, this is Eli. Do you remember? The guy from yesterday, from the Les Halles?"

I sat up straight as if I'd been struck by lightning. Of course I remembered. It didn't happen all that often that someone asked for my number and then actually called.

"H-Hi," I said while sweating bullets, because I was about to have a phone conversation with someone who liked me—*in English*! "Sure, I remember. You found my number in the phone book."

My ability to have a conversation in English at that time was very limited, which is why Eli talked the most. He told me how he was originally from Israel, now working in Düsseldorf for Vodafone in IT; he told me what he thought of Germany, how it was different from Israel, and eventually if I wanted to go out with him this evening.

"I know a great restaurant near the port. It's Mongolian. Have you ever gone to a Mongolian restaurant before?"

"Ehm, no," I said.

I wanted to say more, be more sophisticated than "Ehm, no," but I couldn't. All the English I had ever learned in school was suddenly too shy to come forward. Which is why Eli took over again.

"Even better," he said. "I'll pick you up around six? Will that work? What's your address?"

I looked at my watch. It was 3:30 p.m. We spent almost two hours on the phone. Two very nice hours. I was ready to spend a few more with him over dinner. As always, I wasn't able to say no to food and apparently not able to say no to Eli.

"Sure," I said. My hands were shaking so much, I almost dropped my phone. "Six it is. I'll text you my address."

On our first date, as planned by Eli, we went to the fancy Mongolian restaurant he had mentioned in the port of Düsseldorf. He came to pick me up from my place and then almost forgot about me because he was so excited to meet Fenja. I'm sure he fell in love with my dog that same day, and I fell in love with him a few days later when I came to his place and he had bought a basket, food bowls, and treats for her. We were now part of his life, and even though it was difficult in the beginning for me to have deep conversations in foreign English, it felt . . . normal. We somehow fit together. It was easy to spend my days with him, like *Arsch auf Eimer*—ass on bucket.

I was ready to see the world, and Eli was ready to show it to me. Together we visited Venice; jumped into the car one day and just drove to Italy. I have a picture of me holding Fenja in my arms and Eli holding both of us in his arms, with Saint Mark's Basilica behind us with its breathtaking Italo-Byzantine west façade. I slept in a tent for the first time in my life because of Eli and knew afterward I never wanted to sleep in a tent ever again.

We drove to Paris. I saw the Eiffel Tower, walked alongside the Champs-Élysées, and almost had a heart attack when Eli dared to take the roundabout of the Arc de Triomphe. He introduced me to snowboarding, he got me on a motorcycle, and he even flew with me to Israel, where we walked the cobblestone streets in Jerusalem and went diving with dolphins.

This was the life I had always dreamed of. Adventurous and bold, but also protected because Eli knew what he had gotten himself into and the limitations that came with it. I had told him early on about my CF, about my transplant and all the problems that came with it. He listened, and most of all, he understood what it meant to have a girlfriend like me. The mother of his best friend had been paralyzed from the neck down, so he grew up alongside her and learned what it meant to live with a handicap. A way bigger handicap than mine. Then his father got sick, had multiple strokes, and was bound to a wheelchair, but that didn't stop him from going on vacations with his parents all over Europe. Same as my condition didn't stop him from living the adventurous life he always wanted.

Together with me.

What I had always wished for—a life—he introduced to me in a way I would have never been able to imagine. With Eli by my side, I truly lived life to the fullest and felt completely healthy and whole while experiencing one adventure after another. It was wonderful.

In the beginning of 2007, Eli and I took our adventure called life even further and moved to Vienna, Austria. Never had I thought I would ever leave Germany behind and live in a foreign country. Even though Austria wasn't as foreign (everyone speaks German in Austria), it was still a huge step for me. Suddenly I was 470 miles away from my parents, 470 miles away from their support, but now I had Eli. We got married in September that same year, and in 2009, we moved from Vienna to the United States. To St. Louis, Missouri—foreign indeed.

At first, I was stressed leaving Europe, leaving the proximity of my transplant hospital in Hannover behind, but quickly realized the care for organ transplant recipients was great in the US, if not even better than in Europe.

The main difference in the US was that most doctors perceived their patients as a partner in crime, not as someone to be bossed around. For the first time in my life, I was asked for my opinion, I was given suggestions and not orders, and I loved it. When I told my new doctors at Barnes Jewish Hospital in St. Louis how I only had one X-ray taken per year, they, too, advised me differently but nothing more. I got advice, maybe a raised eyebrow, but everyone accepted that it was my life, my body, and therefore my decision. I felt comfortable with my new care. Comfortable enough to ask that one very particular question I had so far never gotten a positive answer to:

"Can I get pregnant?" The question itself came mostly from my husband. He wanted to have kids, even though he knew right from the start that a pregnancy was most likely not in the stars for me.

Pregnancies were dangerous for any transplant recipient. Reason being, hormone levels changed drastically during pregnancy and could cause an acute rejection of the transplanted organs. Then there were the handful of medications organ recipients had to take to stay alive, which could have an impact on the fetus. And then, further along during pregnancy, the main reason for concern was the growing of the fetus itself. The unborn baby would squeeze my liver and my lungs upward. My lung function would drop due to limited space. My bowel would be moved around, which presented a higher risk for another obstruction. And even if I could stay clear of all these dangerous complications, could deliver a healthy baby, my life would still be at risk for at least two years afterward.

During any pregnancy, the immune system lowers itself so as not to attack the growing baby. As if the immune system said: "Okay, I will let this one slide." But once the baby was born, the immune system would go back to business, and this time with belligerence. For two years, the risk of having a rejection of the transplanted organs would be much higher than usual, just because of the pregnancy. Just because of a vicious immune system.

"Pregnant?" my doctor asked in return and wrinkled his forehead. "We had one lung transplant recipient who had a baby," he said, "and everything went fine. We never had anyone with transplanted lungs and liver, though. But in general, nothing really speaks against it. You are healthy, your lung function is stable, and we can talk about it with our chief physician if you'd like to."

On my way back home, I stopped on the side of the road and called my husband to tell him the great news. We had found *one* doctor who wasn't absolutely against me trying to get pregnant. One.

After hearing from countless others that it was the worst idea one could ever have, *one* doctor was all I needed to give me the faith to at least consider such an undertaking.

During the following weeks, my husband and I met with the chief lung transplant physician, with a high-risk pregnancy doctor, and with a CF doctor. All of them had the same thing to say: "It's possible, but it's risky. Anything can happen, from rejection of the organs to losing the child and/or the mother too. We strongly recommend against it, even though it's possible."

And that was exactly my problem. Anything could happen, but it didn't have to happen. I could die, I could lose the child, I could get a rejection, I could have kidney failure, a bowel obstruction, a miscarriage—everything *could* happen, but it didn't have to. I could also have the most uneventful pregnancy ever. Nine months ending with a healthy baby in my arms. No one knew what to expect because no one ever had a baby after a double lung and liver transplant. I had only question to answer: Was I willing to be the first?

Before we could come to a decision, we moved from St. Louis, Missouri, to Dallas, Texas. It was 2012. I still hadn't made up my mind if I wanted to get pregnant or not. I was worried about getting pregnant and then dying and looking like the biggest idiot ever. For having lost a healthy life just because I wanted a baby. And what would my parents say? My mom would plant cactuses on my grave if I'd die because I had been too greedy and too damn convinced of my health and abilities.

In St. Louis, I had still hoped to just get pregnant by *mistake*, then at least it wouldn't be my fault if I'd die because of it, but when we arrived in Texas, I knew this was not going to happen. I wouldn't just miraculously get pregnant. I had to decide and then live with the consequences. Simple as that. No one would be responsible but me. And my husband.

In the end, it was the right team of doctors and our belief in the impossible that made us decide to give it a try. My husband had always been convinced I would do fine being pregnant, but he had also never seen me on the brink of death. He only knew me healthy, active, breathing, and resilient. How could he imagine tragedy when I had become a poster girl for health?

I, on the other hand, knew how bad things could get, but same as him, I couldn't imagine tragedy even if I tried. I couldn't imagine dying because I was pregnant. I couldn't imagine any of the really bad complications doctors warned me of. I had worked all these years on my belief in my health—how could I die because of a baby when I knew I was healthy?

"You become what you believe you can become," I said to my husband, and the next morning we made an appointment with our fertility doctor.

We both loved our fertility doctor, Dr. B., from first sight. He was very calm, humble, and transparent. He told us openly about his concerns regarding a pregnancy after a lung and liver transplant and about the many medical concerns there were. Which most of them we already knew. But after he met us and learned that neither myself nor my husband had any illusions about how dangerous our journey would be, he agreed to accept me as his new patient. He examined me, blood was drawn, and I got some homework.

"I have printed two studies for you to read." He handed me a pile of papers. "One study is about women with CF who got pregnant. The other one is about women who got pregnant after a lung transplant. Read through them, and if you have any questions, let me know. Otherwise, we will meet again in a week from now to get started."

The ball was rolling, and it seemed as if there was no way of stopping it anymore. I was on the road to pregnancy. After so many years of considering it, gathering information about it, and fearing the worst, the final decision was made the moment we stepped foot into the office of my fertility doctor.

I felt a little bit like I was being tricked into it, but on the other hand, it felt good to be past the decision-making phase and not having to deal with any hypothetical fears anymore. Now we were in it. No guesswork. From now on, every obstacle would be real.

When we got home, I sat down at the kitchen table and started to read the studies the doctor had given me. I was surprised by what I read.

From the ten women who had gotten pregnant after a lung transplant, only *one* of them had been post-transplant as long as four years. Not a very long time after transplant. I was already ten years post-transplant and therefore a way better candidate for a pregnancy.

Further, half of the women had had one or even multiple organ rejections *before* pregnancy. Two of them had had a rejection during pregnancy.

I would have never considered a pregnancy if I had experienced a rejection before. Never. Maybe I wasn't that crazy and irresponsible after all.

Out of the ten women, three had delivered their baby after thirty-seven weeks of pregnancy. Exactly when the baby wouldn't be considered premature anymore. One woman had even made it to week thirty-nine. Five babies had been delivered too early, and one woman had an abortion. All born babies were healthy. None had developed abnormalities due to the medications the women took during pregnancy.

Reading this, I felt like my pregnancy would be a walk in the park. Only when I read the summary did I get a glance at the whole picture.

And it wasn't pretty.

Compared to kidney transplants who had a 4 percent risk of rejection during pregnancy, CF patients had a 40 percent risk of rejection of the lungs during pregnancy. Two years after delivery, the death rate for kidney transplants was at 13 percent; for CF patients, it was at 30 percent. And the end result looked even scarier. The average pregnancy duration of women with a lung transplant was thirty-four weeks. Sixty percent of the babies were delivered prematurely. Sixty percent weighed under 5.5 pounds, 60 percent had complications, and 13 percent died. And I wasn't just a lung transplant recipient; I also had a transplanted liver.

In the evening, I told Eli about the devastating statistics and asked him to reassure me over and over again that I would be fine. That our baby would be fine. My belief was crumbling. The fear was coming back.

Suddenly it wasn't only me I was worried about. I had a 60 percent chance of delivering too early. If I did, our baby would suffer the consequences. Was our decision still acceptable? Were we right to give it a try? Or were we irresponsible to dare to have such a huge dream?

We didn't find any answers to those questions—maybe there weren't any—but we did decide to keep our pregnancy plans secret. It was difficult enough for me to keep faith, to keep any kind of fear at bay, and I didn't need to hear the fear of all the people around us. Especially not the fear my parents would bury me under if they knew.

For the same reason I also kept my plans secret from my transplant doctors at UT Southwestern, until I was scheduled to take hormones. I had to let them know and I was terrified.

From earlier discussions, I knew the chief physician of the lung transplant department was absolutely against pregnancy. Last time I mentioned it, he proclaimed: "You could die!" followed by "I won't treat you anymore if you get pregnant."

He would have fit in perfectly with my doctors in Hannover.

For a short moment, I was worried. I didn't need his approval to get pregnant, but I did need his expertise in taking care of my transplanted lungs.

"But can I still be a patient of this clinic?" I asked.

To my relief, he nodded.

"Yes, but someone else from the team will treat you. I won't anymore."

I was absolutely fine with that. Screw him.

When I came to see my *new* transplant doctor after my appointment with my fertility doctor, the only female doctor of the lung transplant department came to see me. And because she was a woman, she understood my dream of having a baby a bit better, and was ready to support it, even though she didn't recommend it.

And just like that, I had the perfect team of doctors lined up to make the impossible possible. To have a baby. I felt a huge rush of relief. I felt safe with these doctors taking care of me, and for the first time, I felt 100 percent content with what we were about to try. Or at least 99 percent content with it. Some fear and doubt were always there. Somewhere.

A few days later, I had my first hormone appointment with my fertility doctor. After all the back and forth we had gone through, *the day* was finally here. After hearing from countless doctors it wasn't possible. After dealing with my own fear, we were finally about to take the first step toward pregnancy. The only reason for despair: my husband couldn't join me for this monumental appointment. It was a Wednesday, and he had to work, but who was I not being able to handle a hormone injection all by myself? I didn't need my husband for this, or at least that's what I thought. But when I sat in front of my fertility doctor, ready to get poked, he pulled the rug out from under my feet instead and left me to die.

"Inka . . ." The way he said my name, I already felt the world tilting. "I spoke yesterday with the chief physician of the lung transplant department, and he made me realize it's not ethically justifiable to help you get pregnant. We can talk about a surrogate, but I can't help you to get pregnant."

Bam!

Just like that, everything we had worked on for years was destroyed with one phone call. We were back to square one. No one wanted to help us pursue our dream. Absolutely no one.

I stayed polite. I told him I could understand his hesitation, maybe even his decision, and then got up and left. I couldn't fight anymore. I had fought for so long to get to this point. I had fought not only doctors everywhere, but I had also fought my own fears. I couldn't do it any longer. If the world didn't want to give me as much as a single finger for help, then fuck it. I wouldn't get pregnant. We would buy another dog, whatever. No one could change the world without help. And neither could I.

On my way back home, my husband called to find out how everything went, and I started to bawl. I told him everything the doctor had said, how our dream was done, how I was done, so absolutely done with all of this.

"Okay," Eli said, stepping out of his office on the other side of Dallas. "Send me the number of our fertility doctor. I will call him. I will take care of it." Thank God he wasn't done fighting yet. Not even close.

I stopped somewhere on the side of the road, sent him the number, and drove home. Too depressed to argue with my husband that his doing was complete bullshit. How could he change our doctor's mind? My husband was in IT, no medical background whatsoever, so how could he argue that my transplant doctor was wrong and none of this was unethical?

When Eli came home a few hours later, I almost jumped on him, demanding answers to the question "What did you tell our doctor to convince him to get me pregnant no matter what? And did you manage to convince him?"

He smiled, put down his bag, took off his shoes, and walked like a superstar into our kitchen while I was chewing my lips and pacing forth and back. I didn't know if I wanted to sit, stand, or run.

"I," he began, "didn't tell him anything. I told him to call your old doctor in St. Louis, the one who wasn't against pregnancy after transplant, and get his opinion as well. To ask him if he also thought our doing was unethical."

I looked at him for a moment, trying to understand what he was telling me, and then eventually sat down.

"You told him to call St. Louis?"

He sat down opposite me, still an annoying, smug smile on his face. "Yes, I did."

"That was . . ." I had to think for a second. "That was smart. Really smart. And what did he say? Tell me, tell me."

"Who do you mean? Your old doctor in St. Louis or our doctor here? Because I don't know what St. Louis said. I wasn't on the phone call when they talked, but—"

"Our fertility doctor of course," I almost yelled, reaching my hands over the table to grab his. "I don't care what St. Louis said. I only care if they could convince our doctor to get me pregnant!"

He smiled a moment longer, squeezed my hands, and then nodded.

"They could," he said. "Tomorrow morning, you have an appointment to get your first hormone injection."

"Seriously?" I squeezed his hands in return. I couldn't believe it.

"Seriously," he said, and I started to bawl, again. Only this time, it was tears of joy.

26

Risky Business

Our first trial to get pregnant failed.

Our second trial to get pregnant failed.

I was getting nervous.

"What if I can't get pregnant?" I asked my husband after trial number two. "What do we do then? Steal a kid at the airport? Ask my sister if she wants to get rid of one of hers? Adopt?"

"You'll get pregnant, you just have to give it time." He sighed, not at all fazed by two failed trials. "The more you stress about it, the less the chances. Therefore, chill."

But I didn't want to chill. I wanted to get pregnant. Now. Not in two months, not in a year. Now. I was worried something might happen and postpone us again. I could get sick. I could suddenly have a rejection. My liver could act up again, or my so-far-good-to-go kidneys could require attention.

"I just want to be there already," I told my husband. "To move forward." I was just as obsessed as I had been about the call for new organs years earlier.

"And we will," he reassured me. "Wait and see. The third one will be our charm."

And it was. On March 28, 2013, I got my first positive pregnancy test. My husband freaked out. While I was still on the phone with the nurse who had called to inform me of the (finally) positive test, Eli jumped up and down in our backyard like a mad person, with a huge smile on his face, fist-pumping the air as if he'd won Wimbledon. Thank God we were keeping my pregnancy secret, otherwise he would have chartered a plane to skywrite it over Texas: Inka is pregnant!

"Let's see for how long," I said once I had hung up the phone and joined him in the garden. "Let's see if my body is capable of baking a kid."

It took me till week eleven of my pregnancy to feel what my husband had felt from day one.

I had another ultrasound in week eleven but didn't expect much. So far, I had seen a bean getting bigger and bigger. I assumed I would see the same now. An even bigger bean. Nothing human yet, surely not that early on during pregnancy.

But when the ultrasound technician placed the SonoScape on my belly, it wasn't a bean anymore I saw floating around. It was a tiny human. An actual human being.

"This is crazy," I said, pointing at the screen. "Last time it was still a bean, and now it has tiny arms and legs and even feet and hands."

"You can even see the nose," she pointed out, moving the cursor over a little bump that was definitely a nose.

"Crazy," I said once again because I couldn't grasp what I was seeing. A real baby. A real human being. A real miracle. Growing inside of me. Inside of *me*.

We watched in awe how that little human jumped around like a bouncy ball. Floating up and down, left and right, as if it couldn't wait to be born into our world.

And that's when it hit me: I was pregnant. I was going to be a mom. We were going to be parents.

"My husband will be so sad that he missed this," I said to the technician. "He's in Mexico right now, working."

"Oh," she said, but then patted my arm. "Don't worry. I'll print you a ton of pictures to show him every toe and finger."

"And the nose," I said.

"And the nose," she agreed. "And . . ." She pointed toward the screen where her curser hovered over another tiny bump. "The penis."

We were having a boy.

When my husband came back home from his Mexico trip, we decided to finally tell our friends and family about my pregnancy. I was past the first three months, the risk of a miscarriage was small, and we couldn't keep all the joy to ourselves anymore. We wanted to tell everyone. We wanted to brag.

First, we called my husband's family. Since they had never seen me sick either, they weren't shocked by the news. They knew it was dangerous for me, but same as my husband, they couldn't imagine anything going wrong. Everyone congratulated us, expressed their excitement, and then it was time to call my parents.

"Why don't we let the kid tell them when he's old enough?" I asked to stall us.

My husband ignored me, opened my laptop, and then launched Skype.

"It will be such a great moment." I tried to ignore him too. "We can send him over to Germany when he's like six or seven and be like, 'Surprise! This is your grandson.'"

"Call your parents," he said, pushing the laptop toward me. "You have to tell them, and you will do it now."

While Skype dialed their number, I got more and more nervous. I knew my parents would not be happy hearing I was pregnant and risking my life again. We had talked about pregnancy a million times, and they always expressed their strong opinion against it while I had always agreed with them. And now I was about to tell them I was knocked up. And not by mistake, no, we had worked hard to get to this place. I had done everything to get me into the most dangerous position since my transplant. I was sure they wouldn't be thrilled.

"Inka! What a surprise," my mom said when she picked up.

"Yeah," I said, "unexpected, I know. We wanted to tell you guys something. Is Dad there too?"

"Yeah," my mom said, suddenly hesitant. "He's here. What's going on?"

"Oh, nothing bad." At least I hoped so. "Can you guys turn on your computer? We want to send you a picture and be on the phone with you when you see it."

"Okaaay," my mom said, and we heard them going upstairs where the computer was.

"It'll take a moment," my dad informed me. "Computer is turning on."

"I'll send the picture in the meantime. Let me know when you open it."

We heard someone typing on a keyboard, perhaps my dad logging into their email account.

"Did you get it?" I asked.

"It's downloading," my mom said. "Almost there. Is it a new dog? No, wait, is it an ultrasound?" Then silence.

I looked at my husband, who showed me a thumbs-up and waved at the laptop for me to say something.

"Do you see it?" I asked.

"What is that?" my dad asked in the background. And then my mom: "Here, don't you see that? These are the legs, here are the arms, and this is the face."

Without sitting beside them, I could hear the excitement in my mom's voice. She just couldn't help it. My dad was more hesitant.

"You are pregnant?" He asked the obvious; clearly concerned and scared too.

"Yes," I said. "Already for three months."

I told them everything. Especially emphasized the good care we were in, the precautions that were taken, and exaggerated the support we got from my transplant doctors.

"I can't say this was a good idea," my mom eventually said, "but I'm happy for both of you."

I wasn't surprised by her straightforward assessment of the situation. Only in two years and six months, we would know if it had been a good idea, but I was happy to finally be able to talk to my parents about my pregnancy. Same as my husband. Same as my mom.

My pregnancy, even though special in every way, proceeded like any other normal pregnancy. From time to time, I felt nauseous. In the beginning, I was often worried I might not be pregnant anymore and took about a billion pregnancy tests just to prove myself otherwise. Sometimes I cried without reason. In week twenty-five, I cut a good portion of my thumb off while slicing tomatoes. And sometimes I challenged the love my husband had for me when pregnancy hormones took over.

One difference, though, was my routine visits to my diabetes doctor, my endocrinologist. My blood sugar levels during the pregnancy had to be as close to perfect as possible. If my blood sugar was too high, it would increase the risk of our baby being born too early, weighing too much, being stillborn, or even miscarrying.

I learned a lot during these visits about how to control my blood sugar even better, and how I had to change my diet to accommodate it.

I have never been a healthy eater. I loved everything you shouldn't eat. Pizza, chips, cake, gummy bears, you name it. But during my pregnancy, I couldn't eat high amounts of carbs. Everything I ate, every carb I ate, had to be paired with protein, like a slice of cheese or a piece of chicken. Pairing carbs with protein made the blood sugar rise less high and slower.

I did a very good job. If I had one thing under control during my pregnancy, it was my diabetes, which is why every visit to my diabetes doctor felt like a waste of time. Especially because I always had to wait a long time to be seen. Sometimes a very long time.

I sat already for over sixty minutes in the examination room, waiting for my doctor to come in, when I turned to the last page of the book I was reading, thus marking the end of my entertainment.

I sat for a few minutes longer, looked at posters explaining the pancreas and how insulin worked, but was quickly too upset to wait any longer.

I packed up my things, got into my jacket, and left the room, only to bump into my doctor in the hall.

"Oh, Mrs. Nisinbaum," he said with an apologetic smile on his face. "I was just about to come see you."

"And I was just about to leave because I have been waiting already for over one hour to be seen."

I was angry. Pregnancy hormones or not, this was unacceptable.

"I'm so sorry," he said. "I'm ready now, unless you want to reschedule."

I definitely did not want to reschedule and wait another sixty minutes the next time I was here. I shrugged and followed him inside the examination room. I earned this visit.

At first, I was a bit short with him, as I was still angry, but eventually I calmed down. We talked about my blood sugar levels, how my insulin usage would change further along the pregnancy, and eventually talked about the magnitude of what I was doing here.

"I never had a patient who got pregnant after a double lung and liver transplant," he said. "Not even a pregnancy after a lung transplant."

"Yeah," I agreed. "My high-risk pregnancy doctor believes I'm the first one to have a baby after such a transplant. They are already fighting over who will write an article about it all at UT Southwestern."

He perked up. "An article?"

As of now, it had all been small talk, but my mentioning an article sparked his interest.

"Yes," I said. "Since it's probably the first time, some have shown interest in writing about it."

"Maybe my name could be mentioned as well?" he asked, and I couldn't help but smile.

"Sure," I said. "I'll mention it to my doctor, but only if I don't have to wait an hour anymore to be seen."

At first, he was speechless, but then he couldn't help but laugh.

"Deal," he said, and from that moment on, I never had to wait longer than fifteen minutes to be seen by my endocrinologist.

In week fifteen of my pregnancy, I had the recommended Down syndrome test done. I wasn't eager to have everything tested there was to test, but being the high-risk I was, there wasn't much I could do about it.

The test came back negative, but my high-risk pregnancy doctor wasn't happy. My risk of having a baby with Down syndrome was 3:397. Most women had a risk of 1:10,000.

"We should do another blood test to rule out Down syndrome," my doctor suggested, and Eli and I agreed because we didn't really know what else to do. This was our first pregnancy. Our first time hearing about a Down syndrome test. What harm could it do?

"Okay." We both agreed. We both wanted this worry out of the way.

I should have known from all my hospital and doctor experiences that more tests bring more results and only more worries. I should have done what I had no problem doing when it was about my transplant care. I should have said *no*.

The second test came back, and the potential risk had increased. Now I had a chance of 1:271 to have a baby with Down syndrome.

On our way home, I cried. I didn't want to question the quality of our baby. I didn't want to consider a termination. I wanted to keep the life that was growing inside of me. Even if it wasn't perfect. I wasn't perfect. I was born with a chronic and terminal disease, and here I was, living despite it all.

My husband and I had always said we would terminate the pregnancy if my life was in danger. But talking about it and actually considering it were two different pairs of shoes.

"I'm not giving up this child," I told my husband when we were home. "He is perfect. He is healthy. I just know it."

The same way he had always been convinced I would be fine being pregnant, the same way I was convinced our baby was fine. No matter what the numbers said.

"Let's do one more test," he said, and before I could protest, he added: "To know what we will be up against. If he truly has Down syndrome, I want to be prepared. I want to know what we will get ourselves into. Agree?"

I did agree. If our baby boy had Down syndrome, I wanted to know too. The sooner the better.

The following day, I had blood drawn for a "cell-free fetal DNA" test. The test examines cell material of the baby that's floating around in the bloodstream of the mother. If the test found an abnormally high amount of Chromosome 21 in my bloodstream, the possibility of having a baby with Down syndrome would be around 99.1 percent.

Of course, it took a few weeks for the results to come back, in which I almost went insane, but eventually the results came back negative. No high amount of Chromosome 21 in my bloodstream. We could relax. Though I only truly relaxed once I reached week twenty-one of my pregnancy. The moment when a termination of the pregnancy wasn't legal anymore and my baby safe. Whatever doctors would find now, whatever would happen to me, our boy would be born. With three arms or none. He would get a chance in life. Same as I had.

In the same week, we had another ultrasound appointment, and this time my husband was able to join as well.

“Be ready,” the ultrasound technician said, “he’s going to be huge compared to the last ultrasound.” She was right. Our little boy had grown so much while we had been worried sick.

“Here you can see the heart,” the technician explained, “the rips, the bones of the legs, the brain, the face, and”—the last assurance we needed—“the penis, once again. It’s definitely going to be a baby boy.”

We were excited. Everything was there and everything looked perfect. Finally.

Though when we went to bed that night, my husband looked a bit pale despite the good news.

“What’s up?” I asked, lying down beside him.

“We are really going to be parents, aren’t we?” He looked at me with huge eyes.

“Seems like it,” I said, stifling a laugh. “Just as you wanted us to. And we will be great at it. You’ll see.”

In August, we had to say goodbye to Fenja, my dog. I had hoped she would still be able to meet our little man, but she wasn’t. She had been by my side through so much. Moving out from my parents’ place to live in Oldenburg and starting my psychology degree. The time before and after my transplant. My move to Düsseldorf, meeting my husband, moving to Vienna, and then to America, first St. Louis and then Dallas. But my becoming a mom she wouldn’t be a part of. Just before her sixteenth birthday, we put her to rest.

It felt a bit like closing a chapter of my life. Fenja had been with me when I was still sick and crippled by CF. She had been by my side when I had started to believe in my health and began to live with a different perspective. By becoming a mom, I felt like this journey would be complete. Naturally, the focus would move to our baby boy and away from me being transplanted. I would be a mom first, and only then a transplant recipient. Exactly what I had always wanted. Being normal first, and special second.

Week twenty-six of my pregnancy rolled around, and I had another ultrasound. And again, being monitored as closely as I was, wasn't a blessing but a curse. This time it wasn't the risk of Down syndrome my doctor came up with; it was something completely different.

"It looks as if two main arteries carrying blood away from the heart are reversed," the technician said. She printed a few pictures and left the room to get another pair of eyes.

"What is reversed?" my husband asked when the door shut behind her.

"The heart valves?" I shrugged.

"That sounds bad."

"It sounds like bullshit," I insisted. Not being worried but pissed. Another thing that was supposedly wrong with our baby? Really? I was so sick and tired of it all, especially since there was nothing anyone could do about it. I was in week twenty-six. Even if he turned out to be half alien, there was nothing anyone could do about it. He would be born, one way or another.

Another ultrasound technician came running, looked at the pictures, moved the SonoScape over my uterus, and eventually declared: "All looks fine. Nothing to worry about. But now we will do one ultrasound per week. Just to be sure."

It felt like modern medicine had blessed me and slapped me in the face all at once. More ultrasounds would only mean one thing: more ridiculous findings of what could be wrong with my baby. If I would've had emergency confetti available, I would've choked someone with it.

Two weeks later, we moved from our rental house to our first self-owned American house. It had a room for the baby and a huge backyard, and moving while pregnant was just the best. I didn't carry one single box. I only pointed fingers to where boxes and furniture had to go. God bless pregnancy.

And another two weeks later, it was already the beginning of October, Eli and I sat in our beautiful, new backyard, enjoying the still warm Texas weather when it occurred to me:

"If I'll be pregnant for the whole nine months, we'll be parents in ten weeks."

My husband almost choked on his coffee.

"That"—he was still coughing—"can't be right." He pulled out his phone, looked at the calendar and then at me. "You're right," he said. "Only ten more weeks. We need to do some shopping, or the baby will sleep in a carton box."

The upcoming weekend, I was home alone while my husband went shopping, when the so-long-feared-for problems started. I had a weird pulling sensation on my left side but didn't know what it was.

I googled it in connection with third trimester pregnancy and of course found a reasonable explanation called "pelvic girdle pain." Something that was common during the end of pregnancy due to the growth of the baby. Only problem: you could google about anything connected to pregnancy and find an explanation for it on the internet.

Broken toenail during end of pregnancy? The internet had an answer: *Pregnancy hormones can make your nails weaker and more brittle, causing splits and breaks.*

Appetite for cauliflower during pregnancy? Again, Google was there for you: *Five amazing benefits of cauliflower during pregnancy.*

Believing anything written on the internet during pregnancy? Yes, even for this question you could find answers: *You sort of go down a rabbit hole . . . you're just going to keep on searching* was exactly what I did. Until I woke up the next morning after a sleepless night due to excruciating pain and called my high-risk pregnancy doctor.

The good thing was, I could explain my pain to her so well, she immediately knew what was wrong.

"Inner scar tissue," she said. "The baby is pushing your bowel up, but part of it must be stuck somewhere because of inner scar tissue."

"What exactly is inner scar tissue?" I asked.

"Oh," she said. "It's real simple. Every time someone cut open your abdomen, you developed inner scar tissue, or inner scars. One of these scars has connected your bowel to the outer abdominal wall. That's why it won't move up where the baby is pushing it to."

"Like a knot of hair being stuck in my brush?"

She laughed. "Kind of, yes."

"And what do we do about it?"

"I will call in a pain medicine for you. You can take two pills every four hours. Let's start with that. If it doesn't help, call me back and we'll see what else we can do. Best case scenario, the scar tissue will rip and let go of the bowel. Let's just cross our fingers."

The medicine she prescribed for me didn't help at all. When my husband came back from work in the evening, I sat outside in our garden crying. The constant pain had exhausted me. I wasn't even able to lift one foot without having pain. I wasn't able to stand up straight. I walked like a ninety-year-old grandmother after hip surgery, and I had no idea how I would survive another night like this.

"Let's drive to the hospital." Eli helped me to get in the car, and we were on our way.

When we arrived, he first had to get a wheelchair for me. I wasn't able to walk on my own.

We went straight to labor and delivery, where my doctor was already waiting for me.

I got a drip with morphine that made me woozy but didn't help at all with the pain. Only the second drip with morphine did its trick, and I passed out, finally able to sleep.

It was five in the morning when I woke up again. My husband had spent the night on the sofa right next to my bed, worried, not sleeping, and now exhausted as well, but at least we were told to go back home.

I was still in pain, I still walked like a ninety-year-old, but unfortunately, I couldn't spend the rest of my pregnancy in the hospital getting high on morphine. I had to get home and hope for the best. And that's what we did.

It took about a week before the pain was completely gone, before I didn't pop painkillers every two hours anymore and was able to get myself off the sofa without tears and without a helping hand of my husband. We believed the scar tissue had ripped. Nobody knew for sure, and nobody really cared. I was good again. I was able to move, and the fear of having the baby nine weeks early slowly subsided. Everything was good. I was healthy, the baby was growing—no reason to panic. Until, of course, we had another unnecessary ultrasound.

This time, it was the limbs.

"The femur is too short," the technician said, measuring again the length of our baby's legs, but coming up with the same result. Same for his arms. All his limbs appeared to be too short.

"And what do I do now with this information?" I asked my doctor after the ultrasound. "I'm in week thirty-three. There is nothing we can do about it. Why are we even looking for things that could be wrong if there's nothing anyone can do about it?"

My doctor came up with a few explanations: *to be prepared for any possible complication during delivery . . . science . . . because that's what hospitals do* . . . but I didn't care for any of those. I was so angry. I was so annoyed. And I was so ready to tell them they could shove all their ultrasounds up a place where the sun never shines.

When we were back home, I looked at all the ultrasounds and measurements they had taken before and found out our baby didn't only have too-short limbs—they were shrinking. The femur had been longer in week twenty-nine than it was now in week thirty-three. So much for accuracy. If the baby had too-short legs and arms, we would only know for sure after he was born. The ultrasound measurements were good for nothing.

The next ultrasound didn't find any anomalies, but I also didn't allow them to measure the femur again. Long or short legs, this was my baby, and he would be perfect. I didn't allow any other opinion anymore. Finally.

27

NOAM

I looked like a ripe pear in week thirty-six of my pregnancy.

But my mom didn't care what I looked like. She came over from Germany to see me. It wasn't her first time visiting me in the US, as both of my parents had been here before, but it was the most special visit of all. And after all we had been through together: the waiting time, Christmas 2002, the transplant itself, endless days in Hannover, walking up and down the shopping street, hiding from doctors with mouths full of breakfast, my bowel obstruction my mom believed would be the end of me, the mushroom farm in my head; so many times when we had thought this was it, and now here I was, shaped like a pear, about to become a mom.

Because someone had decided to be an organ donor.

"*Mein Schatz*," my mom said when she walked through the sliding doors of International Arrivals and gave me a long hug. "*My treasure.*"

We didn't say much more; there were no words to describe what we were feeling. My mom patted my belly, shook her head in disbelief, and we drove to our house.

A few days later, we had our baby shower. I was officially in week thirty-seven. If the baby decided to come now, he wouldn't be born prematurely. I had made it. I had reached full term. It was indeed a reason to celebrate.

On December 5, I had another checkup appointment with my high-risk pregnancy doctor. No more ultrasounds were scheduled, but they did a pelvic exam to see if I was getting ready to give birth. My due date was December 11 (the birthdate of my brother Malte), and I could go into labor any day now, but everything looked quiet. I was ready to jump up and drive back home when my mom, who had joined me, reminded me of what my diabetes doctor had said.

"Right." I sat back down and explained. "I saw my diabetes doctor the other day, and he said my insulin usage has come down and that it could be a sign of my placenta shutting down."

"True," my doctor said, waving off his concern. "But only if the insulin usage goes down by about twenty-five percent. Otherwise, there's nothing to worry about."

My mom looked at me, and I looked at my mom.

"It did come down by about twenty-five percent," I said eventually, showing my numbers to my doctor to calculate herself. She came up with the same result.

"Okay . . ." She stood up. "Then we will start inducing right now."

"What?" I stood up too, shaking my head while shielding my round belly with my hands. "Right now?" I knew I had almost nine months to prepare myself for this moment, but I still felt overwhelmed. I couldn't have my baby right now. I wasn't ready, not even close. This was way too sudden, and anyhow:

"I haven't even packed my bag to go to the hospital yet. My husband is at work. I need to go home first, and then I'll come back and we can start inducing." I took a step backward, I needed some distance between me and what my doctor was saying. I needed to go home, sit in our kitchen, drink one last tea *and then* I would be ready to become a mom but my doctor shock her head, leaving no room for negotiations.

"Absolutely not," she said. "We got this far. I won't risk a stillbirth due to your diabetes at the last minute. We are inducing now."

I didn't need to know there was a risk of having a stillbirth due to my diabetes, but her argument worked wonders.

"Okay," I said, my voice shaky and my body monetarily frozen, "you convinced me. We will induce now. I just need to call my husband to tell him to hurry up."

The countdown had started. In a few hours, we would be parents. After thirty-nine weeks and one day, I still felt overwhelmed. I knew what was happening, I knew what I had to do, and I knew what was waiting for me regarding giving birth, but anything that came after birth . . . nothing.

One step at a time, I thought. *Just like before my transplant.*

First, I had to get this baby out. Everything else I could worry about later.

When Eli arrived at the hospital, he looked even more confused than I felt.

"What's happening now?" he asked, setting down my bag and looking for a chair.

"We wait," I said.

"And eat," my mom added. We both had ordered some food from the cafeteria and munched along.

When Eli sat down, he shook his head in disbelief at how my mom and I could eat right then. But he finally started to do what we were doing: wait.

We didn't have to wait for long before my doctor came in again.

"The baby is in distress," she said. "His heart rate is all over the place, and I want to get him out now. I do not want to wait and then perform an emergency C-section. Not with a patient like you."

And just like that, our wait time was over.

At 9:01 p.m., our miracle baby was born. He was angry, small, and perfect.

The nurse showed him to me, but I only looked at his face. I didn't count toes or fingers; I didn't try to see if his arms and legs were truly too short. I didn't care. Our son was born, despite all the obstacles we had to overcome. And my body had made it happen. My body that wasn't working as it should, the same body that had always been malfunctioning, had pulled off the most incredible thing a human body could do: it had baked a child. There might not have been parades in the streets after my transplant, but I was sure there were now.

After our son was cleaned and wrapped in a blanket, he was placed for a short moment on my chest. He truly was tiny—only 5.7 pounds—but his cheeks were still round and ready to be pinched. He had a small nose, red lips, and eyes that remained shut. I could still see the anger of being born so out of the blue on his face by the wrinkles on his forehead. Under the hat was thin, brown baby hair peeking out. I felt his heart pumping, I felt him breathing, I felt his warmth. It was in some ways an alienating experience. I knew my whole being was about to change because of this little creature, and on the other hand, I couldn't grasp how this was my baby, how this was my son, and I was his mother, ready to do anything for him even though we had barely met.

After my transplant, I had always said: "I will never get transplanted again. If I need new lungs, I hope I will have the strength to say no and die instead." I had only met my son for a few minutes, but I already knew I would get transplanted over and over again just to be with him. For the first time, I understood what my parents had gone through with me. Being a parent changed everything.

"We have to take him to monitor his blood sugar," one of the nurses said and took him from me again.

My husband's face popped into my visual field.

"It's just a precaution," he said. "It could be that his blood sugar will drop right after delivery. If it does, they need to stable him."

I nodded and suddenly wanted to do nothing more than take a nap. I felt a little bad for wanting to sleep, but my husband was with our son, my mom was beside me, and I could relax. I had survived. My son was healthy. Everything we had dared to dream of had come true. I could have slept for days, but as everyone knows, once you're a parent, sleep is sparce.

After three hours of observation, our little man was finally brought to me and I could welcome him properly, having him lay on my belly, count his fingers and toes, look at his perfect little face, perfectly sized arms and legs, and try to realize that we were parents.

My donor had not only saved my life, but he had also saved the next generation. Our miracle indeed. Our Noam.

28

NORMAL

I continued my endeavor toward health throughout all the years. I never experienced a rejection of the organs after my pregnancy; I practiced my belief; I banned thoughts of sickness as much as I could; and I backed it all up with exercise. Exercise was my newfound proof of being healthy. Whenever I felt sick, whenever I felt I was losing control over my body, I exercised. It was my trick to convince myself that everything was okay. If I could run three miles, if I could do forty-five push-ups, if I could hold a three-minute plank, I couldn't be sick but therefore healthy. It worked like a charm.

Sometimes I had some twitching on my eyebrow and the fear of having another seizure creep up.

"We gotta go for a run," I told my husband every time that happened, no matter what time of day or night it was. "I have to prove to myself I'm healthy."

He always obliged. No matter the time, no matter the weather, Eli jumped on his bicycle and rode along. Once our sweet Noam was there, he bought a treadmill for me so I could run whenever I felt the need for it without us dragging a kid along in the middle of the night. It worked perfectly. I was as fit as I had ever been before. I felt as resilient and healthy as I had ever felt before.

Until the beginning of 2019.

We were living back in St. Louis, Missouri, when I got a cold. Nothing to worry about at first, but it didn't want to go away. I kept exercising, but at the same time, I kept coughing and I felt congested. But what scared me the most was constantly running out of breath. For the first time since my bowel obstruction in 2003, I wasn't able to fix myself by just being stubborn. I had to go and see my doctors, and they confirmed my biggest fear: I had lost one liter of my lung function. Just like that.

All the fear I had controlled over the years came back with vengeance. Suddenly I didn't feel healthy or resilient anymore. I felt helpless, and death was suddenly an option again. Believing in one's health seemed close to impossible when one wasn't feeling well. And I was no exception.

My doctors were as concerned as I was and scheduled a bronchoscopy to figure out what was causing the loss of lung function. Maybe another fungus? A stubborn virus? Some bacteria that didn't belong in my lungs? Anything that hopefully could be cured with a pill or an IV.

But all the tests came back negative. There was nothing living inside my lungs that didn't belong there.

At first, I was relieved. My lungs were clean. I couldn't have hoped for any better news.

But it's never that simple, is it?

"Since we couldn't find any reason for your loss of lung function," my doctor told me, "we have to assume you are experiencing a chronic rejection of the lungs."

My mouth felt open. My body went numb.

"Th-That . . ." I shook my head and tried to form a more coherent thought. "*That* is impossible." A chronic rejection? How could that be? I was healthy. I believed in my health. And as long as I believed in my health, I was. Wasn't I?

"Unfortunately, it is possible," my doctor said without any doubt in his voice. "And we will treat it as such, like we would treat any chronic rejection. You will have to stay with us for a few days, get IVs to deplete the immune cells that cause the chronic rejection, and hopefully stop your decline in lung function."

"How long is the life expectancy after this kind of diagnosis?" I asked. I didn't care what kind of treatment I would have to endure. I only cared for how long I still had. How much time would I still have with my child?

"The prognosis is not as bad as it may sound," my doctor reassured me. "Today we are able to treat a chronic rejection quite successfully. We aren't helpless anymore. But of course, every patient is different. We'll have to see how your body responds to the treatment and go from there."

"And if the treatment works, I'll get my full lung function back?"

"No." The doctor's voice was absolute. This time with certainty. "The goal of the treatment is to stop the decline in lung function and stabilize it in order for you to still have enough function left to be able to sustain it when the next decline comes along."

When I was back home, I googled *chronic lung rejection* in combination with *life expectancy* and learned as much as nothing. The answers I got were as vague as the ones from my doctor. Some articles left me wondering if I should already order a coffin on Amazon, while others talked about five to ten years. But even though five to ten years sounded better than none, that wasn't enough for me. My son was five. I had vouched to make it until he'd at least be eighteen years old. I couldn't die before that. No way, no how. I needed my confidence, my belief in myself, and my body back. And for that, I needed my husband.

"Tell me once again I will be fine," I said to him that evening.

"You will be fine," he said, then looked me in the eyes. "You have survived so much, you gave birth to a healthy kid—a chronic rejection won't bring you down. I know it. As much as I knew we would become parents."

"The doctor said I won't get my lung function back to where it was." I clang to my fear a little longer.

"You never believe what the doctors tell you, so why now? You just have to do what you always do: be stubborn and get moving."

"You mean running?" I asked. I hadn't even thought of that. "I can't run. I'll be out of breath immediately."

"I didn't say run a marathon." Eli sighed. "Start running slowly to feel healthy again. That's what you've been doing all these years, and that's what I had to keep doing with you all these years. Why stop now? Complications are part of life, not the reason to stop believing in it."

Geez, I hated it when my husband was right. Two days later, I signed up for a half-marathon in Chicago in the fall, together with my friend Yukari. When I arrived at the hospital the next day to start my IV treatment for my chronic rejection, I came with my running shoes in tow and asked my doctor, "I can go running outside when I'm off the IV, correct?"

He looked at me as if I had lost my mind, blinking rapidly.

"Can you repeat that? What do you mean by 'running'?" he asked.

"I mean running," I said. "I'm signed up for a half-marathon in the fall. Gotta start my training or I won't make it."

He looked at me again for a moment, and then he laughed and laughed. I had definitely been the first patient who came in for treatment of chronic lung rejection and had to train for a half-marathon.

"Sure," he said eventually. "You can start your training. Just let the nurses know when you leave, stay on hospital grounds, and if anyone asks, I never knew about it."

It was tough starting to run again. First, my body was exhausted from the IVs I got every day. Second, my lungs were truly in bad shape. I had to start very slowly. For the first weeks, I only ran two minutes and then walked two minutes. I wasn't able to do more than that, and it often felt impossible to be running a half in the fall, but I felt the possibility again to survive all this. My stubbornness was back. My belief in my health was growing again, and soon I was determined to show my doctors how wrong they had been by getting all my lung function back. If I had to run ten half-marathons, I'd get there.

On September 29, 2019, I crossed the finish line of my half-marathon in Chicago. Hand in hand with my friend. We had run it in just under two and a half hours. Exactly what we had aimed for.

After we were awarded the biggest finisher medal I had ever seen, I lay in my friend's arms and cried. I wouldn't die after all. I would stay alive and be with my kid because I had just run a half-marathon after being diagnosed with chronic lung rejection. A fucking half-marathon.

I felt incredibly healthy at that moment. I felt like there was indeed nothing I couldn't do if I set my mind to it. Nothing.

It took me overall a full year to get all my lung function back, but I did it. Modern medicine, exercising, and my stubbornness made it possible. And once I was able to breathe again, my belief in my health came back. This time as strong as never before. And then COVID-19 hit, and fear ruled the world. This time not only my world, but everyone's world.

Fear had always been a huge part of my life. It had always been the greatest motivator to try another therapy, take another medication, get numerous chest X-rays done, take countless ultrasounds during pregnancy, and overmedicate rather than under. I had freed myself of some of those fears, but of course had never been immune to fear itself. When COVID-19 hit, I didn't gas up my car anymore—my husband did that for me. I didn't go shopping anymore—my husband did. I carried hand sanitizer around with me wherever I went, and any activities we went to with the kid were held outside and outside only, where I felt safe. But eventually, over the course of the first COVID-19 months, I decided for myself that this was not the way I wanted to live my life.

Despite all I had been through, I still had a shorter life expectancy than others and therefore couldn't afford to put my life on hold for who knew how long. I had to live *now* because I didn't know if later would exist for me. I had to make the best of the time I had, the best of the time I had *now*, during COVID-19, because there was no guarantee for a time after.

Instead of staying home all summer barricaded in our basement, we decided to do a road trip with our camper. We would sleep in our own mobile home. We would cook in our own mobile kitchen and not sit in restaurants, and we would be outdoors most of the time and therefore be as safe as possible while still making memories. I felt good about that plan. There was a little bit of fear, but not too much.

Therefore, for the duration of two weeks, we drove from Missouri through Kentucky, Tennessee, Alabama, and all the way to Florida, where we stayed a few nights right by the white sandy beach of Navarre.

On our way back, we stopped in deserted New Orleans, drove through Mississippi and Arkansas, and made it all the way back to

Missouri. We used tons of soap and hand sanitizer. The main item of every load of laundry I washed during our trip was face masks. I exercised obsessively, every day, to stay healthy and to prove to myself I still was. If we ate out, we sat on the restaurant's patio, never inside, and every child-friendly activity we participated in was outdoors, always outdoors. It was the most wonderful vacation during the most worrisome time.

I was glad when we were back home, still healthy despite all our travels, and somewhat safe again. But I was also glad I had taken the risk of having a vacation together. If COVID-19 would get me now, my son would be able to look back on two wonderful and exciting weeks he had had with his mom. He would be able to look back on time filled with laughter, excitement, adventure, and beauty—wonderful memories instead of just empty time spent at home. Same as I. To me, it had always been the memories that counted, not the time. The memories I had made would be the ones that would defy death when he'd come for me, not the time I had been able to run away from him.

The year 2020 ended, and we were able to look back on a year of time well spent. Even though I broke my arm four times in August. Two compound fractures, followed by a complicated operation, and months of physiotherapy and limitations. I broke it while playing tag with second and third graders, not skiing.

Life was just like that.

Normal.

About the Author

Inka Nisinbaum has a knack for beating death. She became the first woman to give birth to a healthy baby after receiving a double lung and liver transplant. No matter what's thrown her way—like cystic fibrosis, chronic lung rejection, or cancer—Inka fights back with snark, cuss words, and her favorite companion: stubbornness. She has also translated subtitles for *MacGyver*, ran two half-marathons, and raced new and vintage cars for 2000 km Durch Deutschland. When she's not defying all odds, she's writing stories that make room for miracles. She is the author of *Ich Bin Noch Da*, *Emails vom Tod*, and *Emma und Sam*. Inka lives in Colorado with her always-cooking husband and her all-around athletic son. *The Anomaly* is her debut English memoir.

Connect with the Author

Instagram.com/inkanisinbaum

Leave a Review

If you enjoyed *The Anomaly*, will you consider leaving a review on your platform of choice?

Reviews help authors find more readers like you. Thank you!

Afterword

All the negative experiences I had at Hannover Medical School in Germany are true. But what's also true is that I owe my life to the doctors in Germany. They are the reason I'm still here today. Their courage to undertake another double lung and liver transplantation, after the previous one was not successful, saved my life. Even though not everything went smoothly post my transplant, I will never forget that this miracle started with all of you—transplant surgeons, transplant doctors, and transplant nurses.

Thank you!

www.ingramcontent.com/pod-product-compliance
Lightning Source LLC
Chambersburg PA
CBHW070248130726
48054CB00022B/154
* 9 7 9 8 9 9 5 9 9 3 5 0 6 *